yoga

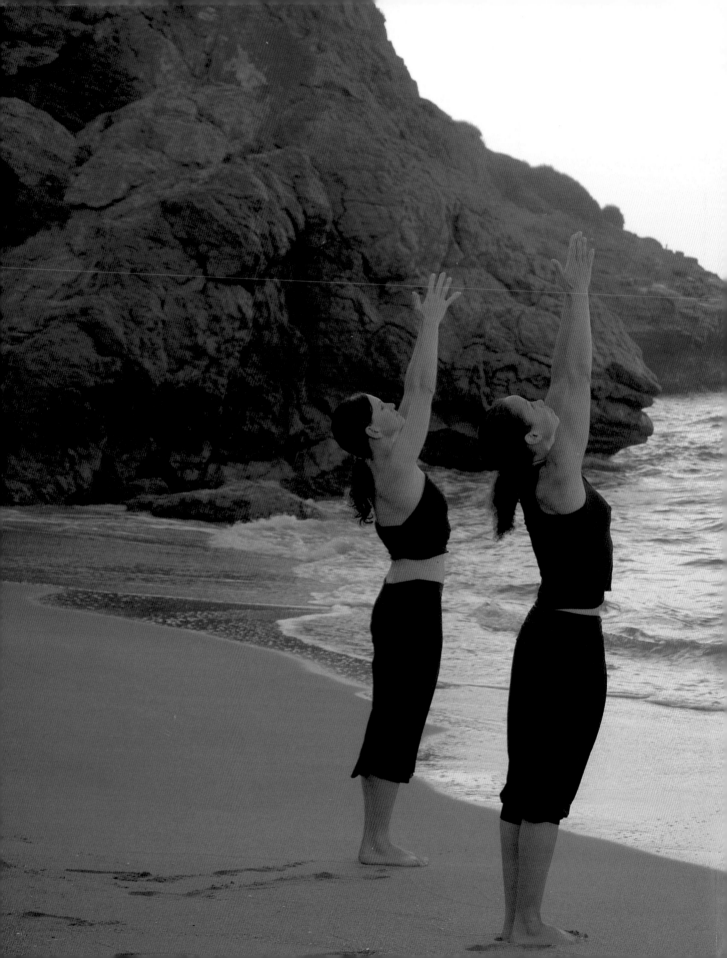

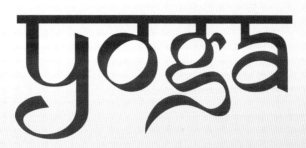

yoga

THEORY AND PRACTICE FOR BEGINNERS AND ADVANCED STUDENTS

Inge Schöps

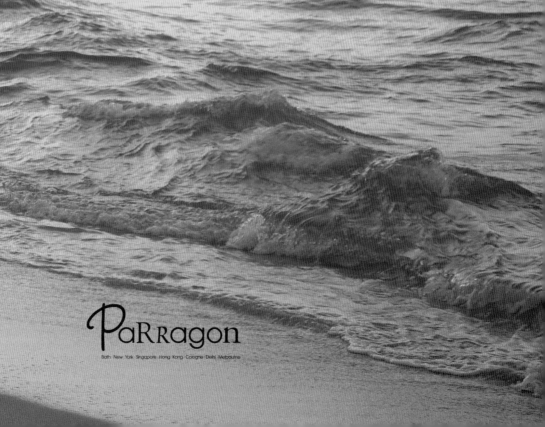

PaRragon

Bath · New York · Singapore · Hong Kong · Cologne · Delhi · Melbourne

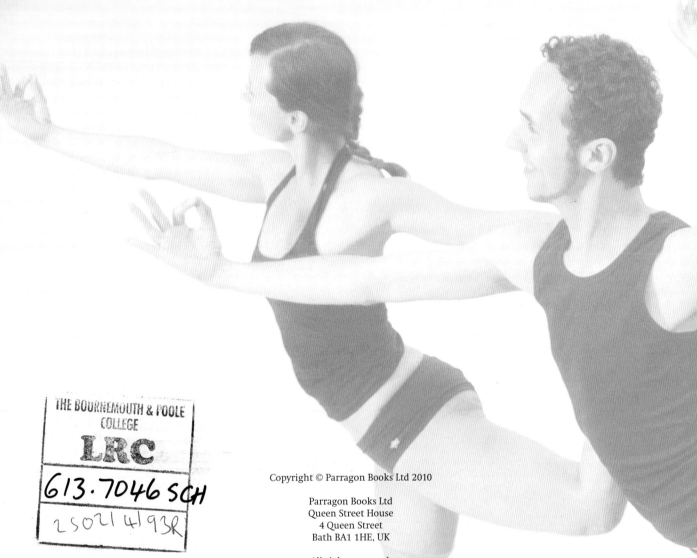

Copyright © Parragon Books Ltd 2010

Parragon Books Ltd
Queen Street House
4 Queen Street
Bath BA1 1HE, UK

Author and editor: Inge Schöps, Cologne
Photography: Günter Beer, Garraf
Models: Nicole Bongartz, Eduardo Castro-Neves, Constanze Handmann, Ijeoma Ollawa,
Dulce Jiménez-Sedano, Cologne
Design, layout and typesetting: Workstation GmbH, Bonn
Editing: Kirsten E Lehmann, Cologne
Technical editing and exercise sequences: Lord Vishnus Couch, Cologne
Proofreading: Kristina Bönig, Cologne

English-language edition produced by Cambridge Publishing Management Ltd
Translators: Michele McMeekin, Tess Pike

ISBN 978-1-4075-6402-9

Printed in Indonesia

NOTICE
The information contained in this book has been carefully researched but is not intended to be taken as a replacement for medical advice.
Any person who is ill or requires medical attention should consult a qualified physician
before starting the exercises described in this book.

CONTENTS

INTRODUCTION
Yoga: The promise of freedom

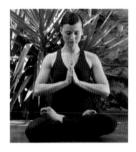

Ancient teaching

Yoga is one of the oldest teachings and philosophies that takes a holistic approach to the individual, focusing on the body, mind and spirit to create harmony and unity. The practice of yoga is based on at least 3,500 years of collected knowledge of how the body is built and how the mind works. This involves exploring a whole host of possible barriers to achieving harmony of the body, mind and spirit, and developing effective exercises to permanently alleviate or remove these obstacles, thereby achieving peace of mind.

Yoga disciplines

However, the term 'yoga' also incorporates the disciplines that can be used to arrive at this state. The essential elements are: practising the physical postures of yoga, or asanas, controlled breathing, or pranayama, meditation, chanting and reading ancient scriptures.

Depending on the personal disposition and individual preferences of the practitioner, priority can be given to different disciplines. However, all paths lead to the same goal: freedom.

yogaścittavṛt-tinirohdhah

Yoga is when the turnings of the mind are stilled. (Yoga Sutra 1.2.)

State of yoga – the still mind

Yoga is a state in which the body, mind and spirit are in unity (the word 'yoga' comes from the Sanskrit *yuj*, to bind together). This goal is timeless, which makes yoga as vital and modern today as it was thousands of years ago. When the state of yoga is achieved, the mind is still and the perception clear, resulting in a feeling of unity and happiness.

The goal – great freedom

Yoga assumes that each individual is prevented from acting in a clear, conscious and insightful way by physical and mental conditioning, mind patterns and misconceptions. The aim of yoga is to be liberated from these afflictions and to achieve inner peace – the basic prerequisite for freedom from internal and external constraints.

The positive effects of yoga

Whether it is used as a gentle or demanding fitness programme, as a form of treatment, as part of an ethical lifestyle, as a spiritual experience or last – but by no means least – as a source of pleasure, there are plenty of reasons for taking up yoga. Yoga is for anyone of any age, and can be practised at any time, wherever you are.

Yoga:
- *improves stamina, strength and flexibility*
- *increases vitality and energy*
- *leads to an improved awareness of the body*
- *reduces tension and pain*
- *delays the ageing process*
- *alleviates complaints of old age*

- *leads to inner peace and harmony*
- *helps build up resistance to stress*
- *improves quality of life and mental well-being*
- *develops stamina and concentration*
- *improves the ability to focus and provides mental clarity*
- *harmonizes the body, mind and spirit*
- *opens up new perspectives and approaches to life*
- *helps to identify and overcome unwanted cravings and habits*
- *boosts self-confidence and self-awareness*
- *goes hand-in-hand with an ethical lifestyle*
- *allows for spiritual development.*

'Regular yoga practice helps you to confront the hustle and bustle of everyday life calmly and steadily.' (B.K.S. Iyengar, b.1918, internationally recognized authority on yoga)

Freedom means completely different things to different people. For many it is a feeling of happiness, an inner peace and independence from external demands, of self-awareness or enlightenment. For others, freedom means feeling at one with nature, connecting the individual to the great totality, the cosmos or the divine. Yet others see freedom as being a mixture of all these things. Yoga has a term for this: *samadhi*, meaning 'the absolute'.

The inner path

Whatever is felt to be the absolute, yoga always follows an inward path. It requires you to explore and get to know yourself. Yoga is an inner composure that demands and at the same time promotes attentiveness and consciousness. By following this path, yoga offers a whole host of beneficial effects that enrich everyday living – even if you ultimately fail to achieve the absolute.

As well as providing a whole range of positive effects, the practice of yoga is fun and brings pleasure into your life.

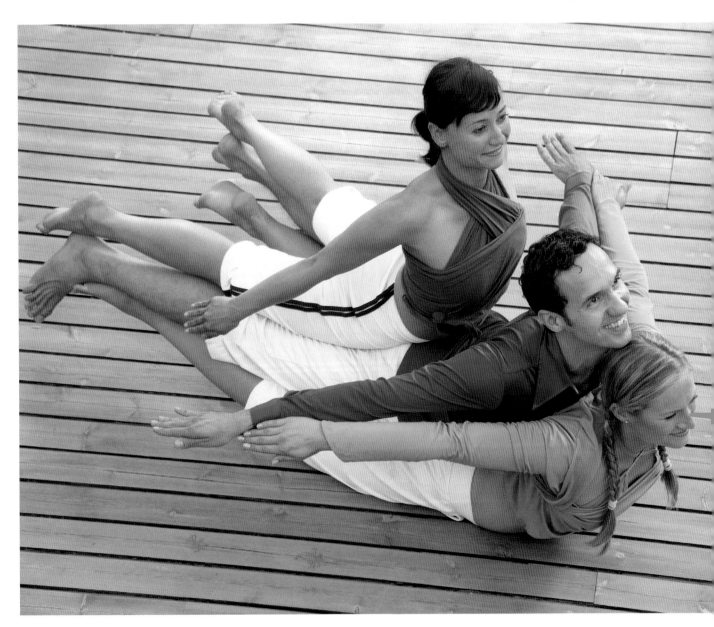

About this book: A practical companion

Yoga is made up of 1 per cent theory and 99 per cent practice and experience.

Yoga is something you can experience for yourself. Most people take the practical approach to yoga by performing the physical exercises, called asanas. The wonderful thing is that yoga produces immediate results!

This book not only offers an introduction to the history and philosophy of yoga – from religious yoga through Patanjali's Yoga Sutras and the emergence of Hatha Yoga, to modern-day yoga practices – it also describes the asanas in conjunction with controlled breathing techniques (pranayama) and meditation.

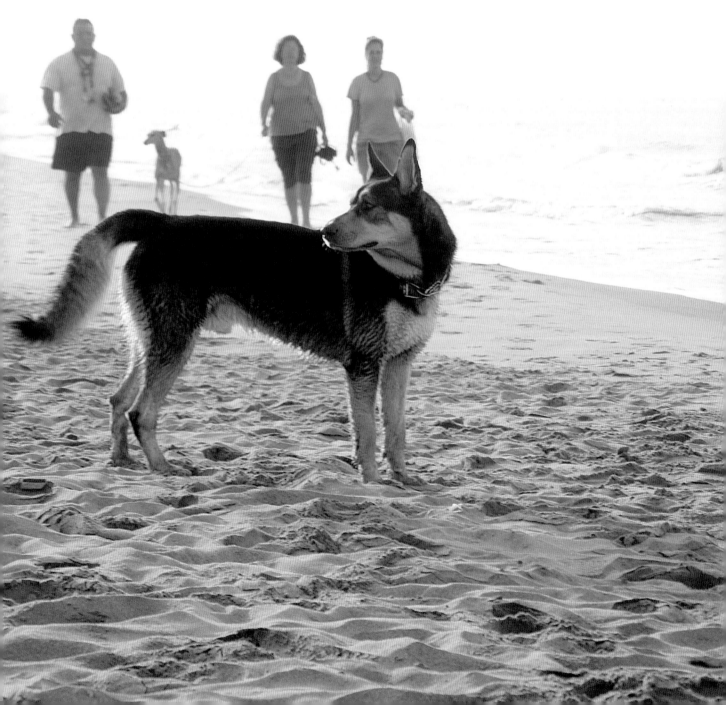

From preliminary to advanced practices

The book is aimed at both the beginner and advanced student and is a companion for those wishing to develop their yoga practice. This means that both the basic postures and also more complex positions are shown. However, it does not claim to be exhaustive, as there are thousands of asanas and countless variations.

The asanas chosen for this book – over 120 of them plus different variations – mainly cover those taught in most yoga classes. Every one of the asanas presented here includes photographs and a detailed description. Where necessary, in addition to a step-by-step guide, simpler alternatives are shown for the beginner, while more complex options are provided for the advanced student or those who have mastered the basic techniques. This allows the essence of each asana to be made clear, so that it can be understood and practised in all its forms.

The same applies to the principal breathing and meditation techniques in the later chapters on pranayama and meditation. In the final section of the book, a series of exercise sequences is presented; these are intended for different times of the day and for different levels, and can be practised at home or on the move.

A good teacher is a must

This book cannot replace a good yoga teacher, but it can be treated as a companion to a yoga class. It is always advisable to practise with a certified yoga instructor who will be able to offer support and advice and correct any mistakes.

Have fun on your path to yoga!

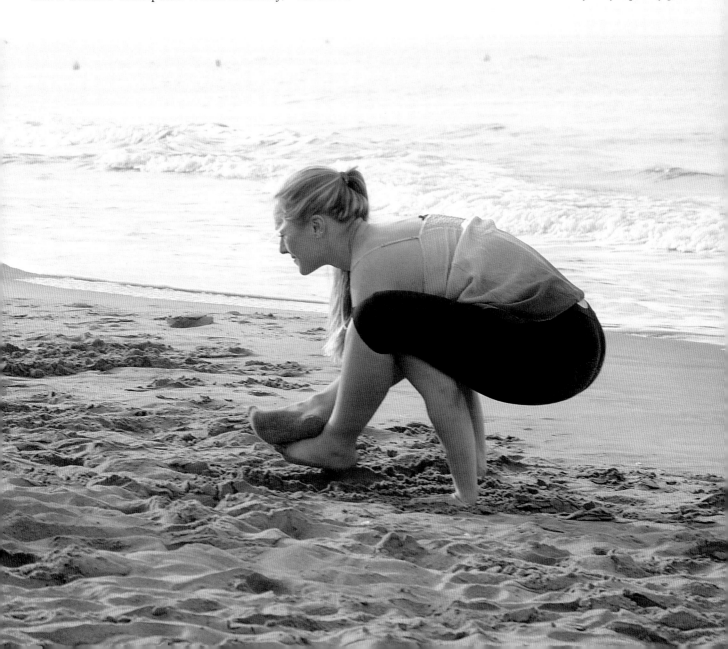

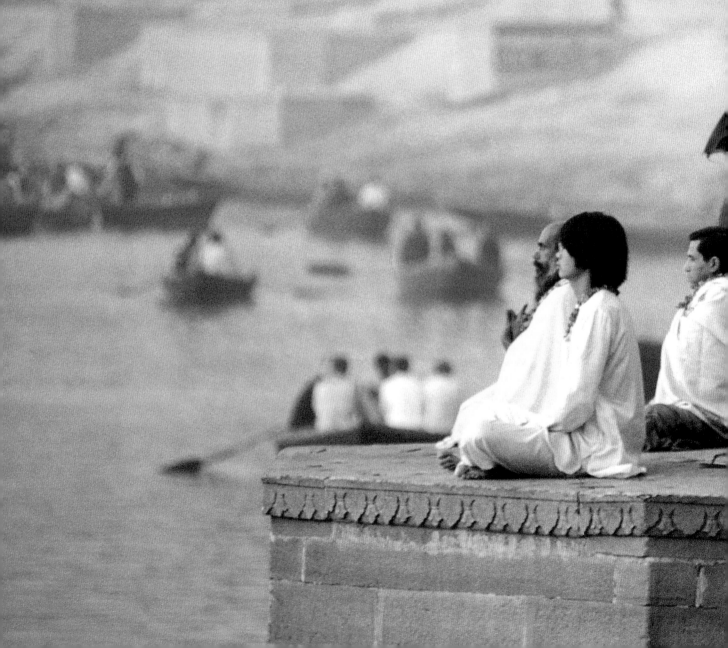

yoga
History and philosophy

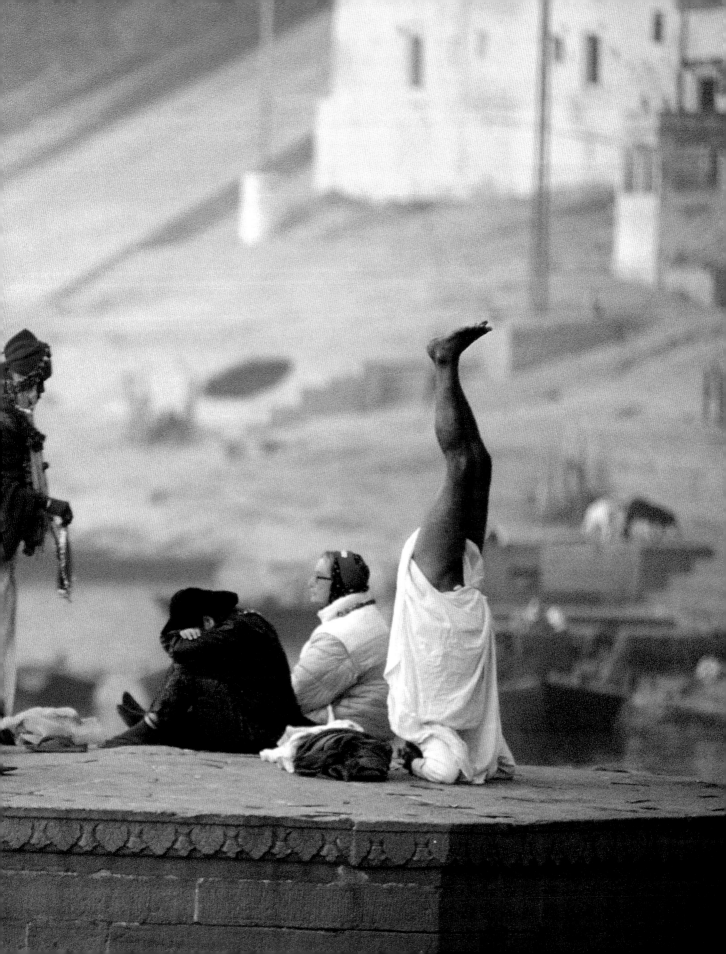

YOGA KNOWLEDGE: THOUSANDS OF YEARS OLD

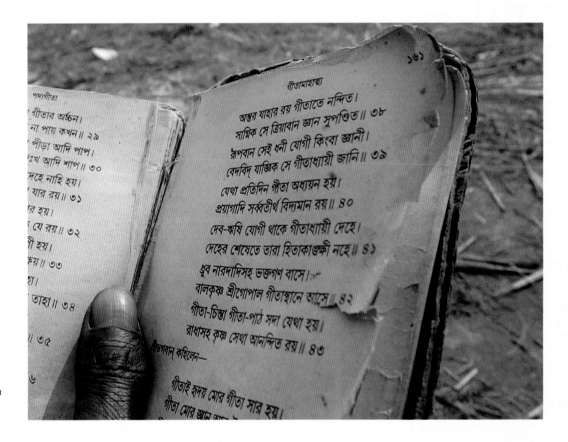

The yogic philosophy of life developed from three ancient Hindu scriptures: the Bhagavad Gita, the Yoga Sutras of Patanjali and the Hatha Yoga Pradipika.

The word 'yoga' derives from the Sanskrit root *yuj*, meaning to yoke, draw with a team of horses, bind together or unite.

Yoga has existed in India for over 3,500 years. In 1500 BC, nomads from Central Asia (Aryans) began to move further into the Indian subcontinent, bringing with them their class, or caste, system, and an intellectual discipline they referred to as 'Yoga'. This included ways of using the mind to restrain the senses and control the body. An image can be used to illustrate this: the intellect is like the charioteer who controls his horses, or five senses, which in turn pull the chariot, or body, to lead it in a particular direction.

The three main yoga traditions

Over thousands of years, three principal lines of tradition have developed in yoga based on different fundamental texts:

1. **Religious yoga** is based on the Upanishads, a collection of texts from around 800 BC, which set out, discuss and comment on the essence of the Vedas, the ancient Hindu writings on religion and philosophy. Another source of Hindu wisdom, the Bhagavad Gita, or 'The Song of God', is also attributed special significance in yoga. It is made up of 18 verses from the Mahabharata epic, which, along with the Ramayana, form the national epic that came into being around 500 BC. This great collection of texts represents the historical knowledge.

2. **Classical-Philosophical yoga** is based on Patanjali's Yoga Sutras (created some time between 200 BC and AD 200), which are often referred to as the fundamental texts of yoga. These sutras (literally, 'threads') describe how the intellect works and open up a way of stilling the mind and gaining knowledge of oneself and the world.

3. **Hatha Yoga** is based on the Hatha Yoga Pradipika (written between AD 800 and 1200), which is in some ways a manual on Patanjali's Yoga Sutras. It describes how to train the body, so that it can be used as a means of enlightenment.

The Bhagavad Gita, the Yoga Sutras of Patanjali and the Hatha Yoga Pradipika formed the basis for developing the central concepts of yoga's philosophy of life. All the later works on yoga are in some way rooted in one or other of these writings and the yoga practised today often combines one or more traditions.

Yoga is not a religion

Although yoga's roots are closely linked to Hindu culture, yoga should not be misinterpreted as a religion. While the fundamental historical texts repeatedly refer to an undefined spirituality, this is actually a method of controlling the body through the mind and in this sense it is a sort of doctrine of self-discovery that is detached from any particular religion or belief system. The path of yoga can be taken by those seeking to develop their body and mind, irrespective of religious convictions. Many millions of people of all different faiths – Christians, Hindus, Muslims, Jews – as well as agnostics and atheists practise yoga.

Those who have difficulty with the notion of a 'divine consciousness' can replace this with their own meaning to express anything that is beyond an individual's own powers – life, nature or the universe.

'Yoga is not asking you to believe in anything in particular; yoga is saying "Experience things!" Yoga is not a belief. It is the penetration of one's own existence.' (Osho, 1931–90, also known by the name Bhagwan, controversial scholar and philosopher)

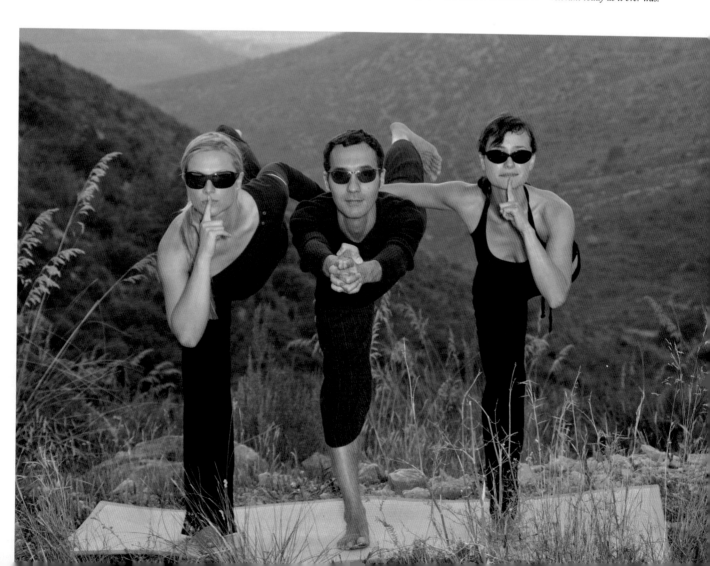

Yogis in the modern world. Although yoga is based on ancient knowledge, it is as relevant today as it ever was.

YOGA WITH A RELIGIOUS INFLUENCE
From the Vedas to the Upanishads

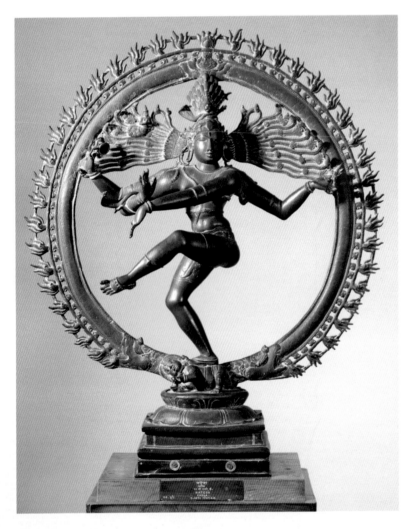

Shiva, one of the three most important Hindu gods, stands for change and transformation and is therefore the god of the yogis. As in this case, he is often depicted as a dancer (bronze statue, India, 12th century).

the Brahmins during deep meditation, and as such could not be changed.

Sacrifices and ecstasy rituals were used to appease the gods and to guarantee the success of the sacrificial offerings. Over the centuries, these rituals became more complex and the efforts made by the practitioners grew and grew. So-called fakirs – members of religious Hindu orders – have tried right up to the present day to detach themselves from the material world (and to placate the gods) by practising extreme asceticism and yoga.

Yoga – a practical approach to self-discovery

As the religiously influenced sacrifice rituals and yoga practices became increasingly extreme, they started to be called into question. The first transcripts of the Vedas in around 1000 BC meant that knowledge that had hitherto been the preserve of the Brahmins was for the first time more widely accessible (even though there was still only a small minority of readers), providing a basis for discussion and reflection. Study of the Vedic texts by teachers and pupils touched upon the fundamental questions of humanity and the world. They were summarized in the Upanishads in around 800 BC, which can be regarded as the essence of the Vedas.

The Vedas – the oldest collections of scriptures on the spiritual, philosophical and scientific knowledge of India (before 1000 BC) – tell us that yoga was practised from early times in the context of religious sacrifices and mystical ecstasy rituals. The transmission of knowledge was the responsibility of the highest caste within society, the Brahmins (priests and sages); this involved a close teacher-pupil relationship with oral recitation, whereby knowledge was passed on through instruction. The words of the Vedas were seen as a divine revelation, which had been received by

The Upanishads contained a wealth of commentaries, which were in turn discussed over the centuries. They developed the central philosophical idea that everything is one and consequently God is in everything and everything is in God. This new world-view meant that the sacrifice rituals once influenced by religion became superfluous – the self was now interpreted as divine. The focal point of practical yoga also shifted during this time, concentrating on recognizing the true self, or Atman, through meditation.

The gods of Hinduism at a glance

In ancient times, the pantheon of Hinduism was populated by countless gods, each with clearly defined responsibilities. There was the god of thunder, the god of the sun, the god of wind and many more besides. From around 1000 BC, religious beliefs focused increasingly on the so-called Trimurti, or trinity of Brahma, Vishnu and Shiva.

Brahma, the creator of the universe, is usually depicted as a paternal figure, but because he leaves the god Vishnu to oversee the fate of all that has been created, he is seldom worshipped.

Vishnu, the world's custodian, is full of sympathy and cares primarily about people. As a result, he is worshipped deeply and passionately and has a large following. Images often depict him lying on the snake Adisesha, which protects both him and the world with its 1,000 heads and is the keeper of all treasures. In order to help all creatures, Vishnu has left his comfortable position nine times and returned to this world. Rama, Krishna and Buddha are probably his best-known incarnations. Legend has it that Vishnu ordered his snake, Adisesha, to be reincarnated as Patanjali (see pp.20–31), so that he could bring a practical form of yoga to man.

Shiva, the destroyer, symbolizes dying, death and change. He destroys everything that Brahma has created, including illusions, ideas, models and customs. This makes him the god of the yogis too. He makes space for the new and enables transformation to take place. He is frequently depicted with a trident and blazing hair or as a dancer.

Stone door lintel depicting the trinity of the Hindu gods Brahma, Vishnu and Shiva (India, 12th century).

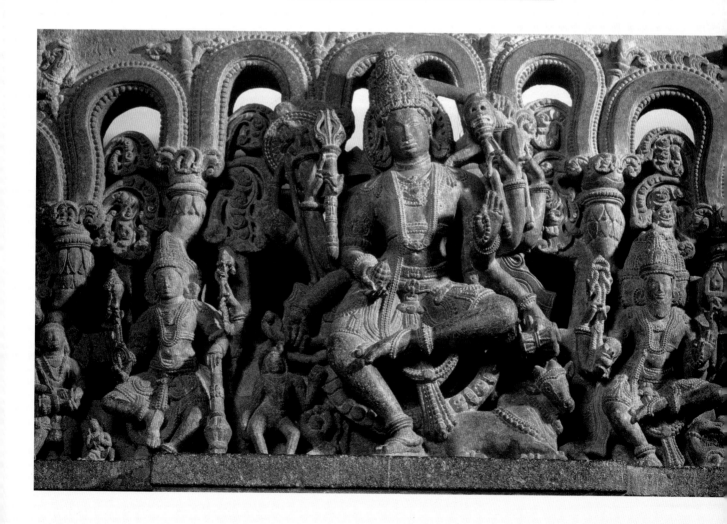

Yoga as an escape from the eternal wheel of reincarnation

Not every caste promises life is a bed of roses.

The folklore and legends collected in the Mahabharata and the Ramayana gave members of all castes (those who could read, at least) previously denied the knowledge and practice of religious rituals access to a spiritual system. This had formerly been the exclusive preserve of men belonging to the top three castes, insofar as they could afford it, as the Brahmins were well paid for passing on their knowledge of the connection to God.

The Song of God

One of the fundamental sources in which yoga is described as the path to knowledge and the redemption of man is the Bhagavad Gita, or 'The Song of God', part of the Mahabharata, which appeared around 500 BC. In it, Krishna, a reincarnation of the god Vishnu, explains to the war hero, Arjuna, that anyone, irrespective of the caste he was born into, can follow the path of yoga and use the methods and techniques to find Atman, the true self and divine being within.

The path of yoga offered each individual a system of techniques and methods of achieving self-awareness and connecting with the divine within their own being. In this way, everyone could influence their fate and take responsibility for their life, so that they were no longer dependent on the help of Brahmins to escape the 'eternal wheel of reincarnation' according to Hindu beliefs.

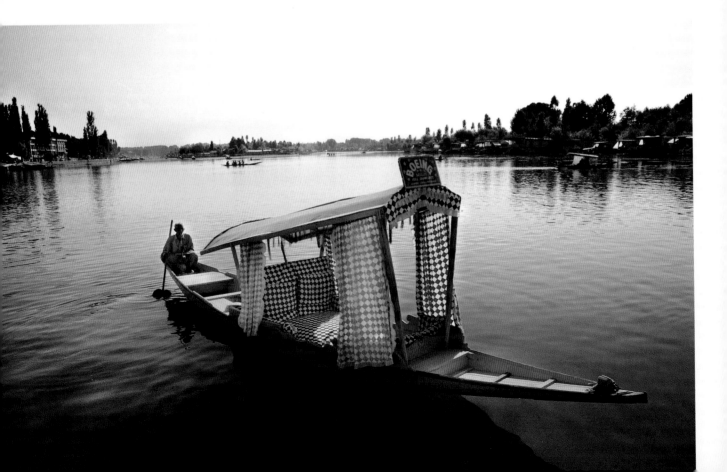

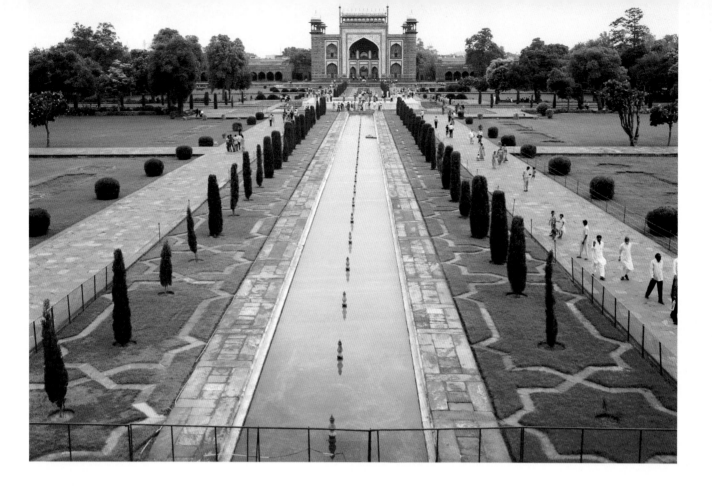

Dharma:
The all-embracing law of the world

Indian culture is based on an all-embracing law of the world known as Dharma (which is Sanskrit for 'purpose', 'law' or 'duty'). According to this, every individual has a destiny to fulfil and everyone has the task of discovering what has to be done in their lives, in order to embrace their own nature – to know Atman, the divine consciousness within. This means that every being has rights, obligations, characteristics, boundaries and capabilities according to their nature.

This is also the basic assumption underlying the Indian caste system. Everyone is born into a particular caste, which is the result of the Karma, or actions, collected in the previous life. Consequently, everyone can fulfil their duty, their Dharma, within the framework of their capabilities, thereby improving their Karma and moving into a higher caste in the next life. The aim is to unite the self (Atman) with the universal spirit, or Brahman, and to one day escape the eternal wheel of reincarnation.

The law of Karma

The law of Karma, the cycle of cause and effect, also creates the ethical foundation of yoga. According to this, every action has consequences, whether in this life or the next. This means that everyone is responsible for their actions and can influence the result of these within the realms of their capabilities, so that they enjoy good Karma or have to suffer bad Karma sooner or later.

If the Dharma, or purpose, of a person's life is fulfilled, they will have a good chance of improving their Karma and moving up a caste in the next life, thereby improving their living conditions. The path leading to this can be a tortuous one, however.

Buddhism and Jainism

Two other religious–philosophical systems developed in India in around 600 BC – Buddhism and Jainism. At the heart of both is the law of Karma and reincarnation.

THE YOGIC VIEW OF THE WORLD THROUGH THE AGES
Universal consciousness

The notion of a universal consciousness was already being developed in the teachings of the Upanishads. Early yoga had numerous names for this state of consciousness – Brahman, Purusha, Ishvara, Atman, to name but a few – and it used these to denote anything associated with divine consciousness. This universal consciousness embraced the seeing, the seen and the act of seeing in equal measure, and manifested itself both in the external world and in the soul, in other words, in Atman, the divine consciousness within each individual being.

Truth and illusion

In around 400 BC, an Indian school of philosophy called Samkya developed a new way of looking at universal consciousness: this is reality and it exists forever. Everything else – referred to as Maya – is simply an illusion concealing reality. Consequently, the world as it is perceived is simply a reflection of the illusion that is created in the mind and not a manifestation of divine consciousness. According to these teachings, nature, all living beings, bodies, intellect and emotions are separate from the divine. They do not require any special attention, because they are part of the illusion and are constantly changing.

Purusha and Prakriti – the dual view of the world

This radical view of the world was not entirely shared by subsequent generations of yogis, who practised yoga on the basis of Patanjali's Yoga Sutras (see pp.20–31). They took the more global view, which corresponded to the dualist view of the world. According to this, the world is divided into universal consciousness (Purusha) and individual consciousness (Prakriti). Purusha is the divine entity that sees the truth and has a cosmic consciousness of immortality. Purusha is enduring, timeless, real and unchanging, somehow representing the primordial state, which manifests itself in Atman, the divine essence of each person. In contrast, Prakriti is the changeable nature, the outer shell, which consists of everything that can be seen and experienced. This matter manifests itself in three forms, referred to as 'gunas'.

Gunas – the qualities of nature

Everything that constitutes Prakriti has three fundamental forms, or gunas:
Sattva is characterized by lightness, purity, balance, clarity and equanimity;
Rajas is characterized by activity, impulsiveness, restlessness, passion, growth, evolution and change;
Tamas is described as darkness, heaviness, resistance, ignorance, sluggishness and inertia.

Prakriti is therefore always a combination of these three qualities, with one or other prevailing. A yogi seeks to achieve sattva in all his thoughts, deeds and feelings. Pure sattva cannot be achieved in the material world, but yoga techniques can be used to mitigate the negative influences of tamas and rajas on the body and mind. Tamas is overcome by rajas and rajas by sattva.

Identification with Prakriti is a constant source of distress, due to its erratic nature. Yoga seeks to explore everything material, but without becoming a prisoner of it, with a view to penetrating the essence of universal consciousness or, in other words, to achieving unity between Purusha and Prakriti.

Since time immemorial, yogis have been exploring the notion of universal consciousness through meditation (gouache on paper, India, 19th century).

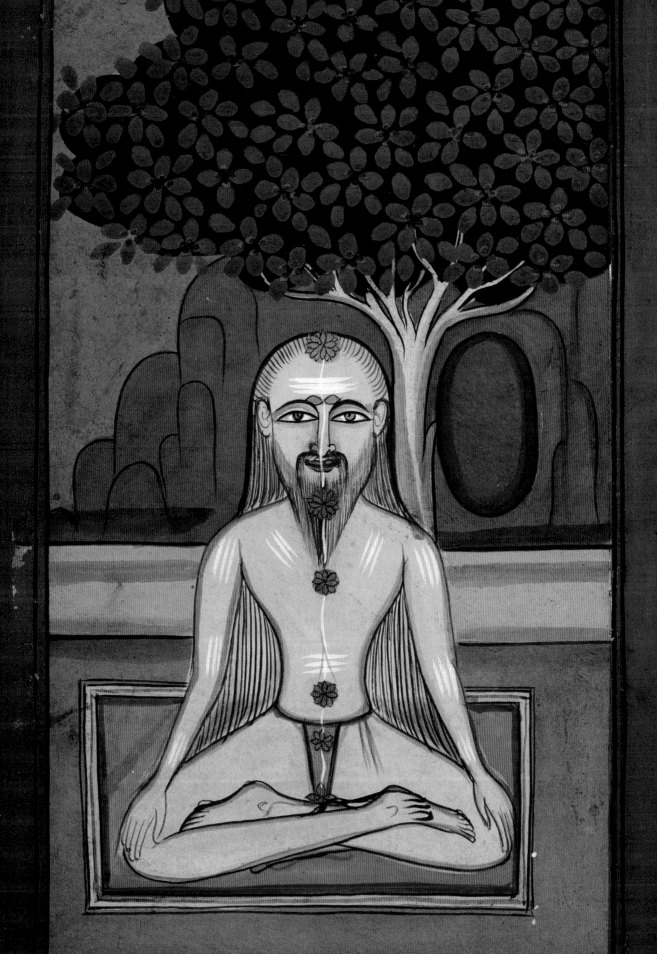

PATANJALI'S YOGA SUTRAS
Stilling the mind

The yoga of Patanjali is also called Classical Yoga, Raja Yoga or Kriya Yoga.

Yoga techniques were systematically summarized for the first time by Patanjali in the Yoga Sutras (from the Sanskrit *sutra*, 'thread') between 200 BC and AD 200. The precise background to their emergence is not known. Whether Patanjali is the name of an individual, a family of Brahmins or a union of magi/philosophers is still unclear. Legend has it that Vishnu ordered his snake, Adisesha, to be reincarnated as Patanjali, so that she could bring a practical form of yoga to the people.

Philosophy and psychology rolled into one

The sutras, 195 of them in total, were written in short, concise but meaningful sentences. As in modern psychology, they describe how the mind works and the obstacles, difficulties and emotional disturbances that can affect it and stand in the way of self-knowledge and reflective action. Patanjali's Yoga Sutras recommend the so-called 'Eight-Limb Path' as the way to changing the mind positively. Following this path leads to recognition of the causes of suffering and provides the means of avoiding them in future, leaving the way open to self-knowledge.

A 'monkey mind' that jumps back and forth

Samskara: Deep-rooted thought patterns, conditioning and habits, which leave an imprint on the mind and are hard to escape.
Citta: The mind, thought or understanding, which interprets everything that is perceived.

According to Patanjali, one of the mind's fundamental characteristics is that it normally refuses to remain in the here and now. Instead, it jumps about like a monkey from one branch of thought to the next. It is constantly and relentlessly on the move, never focusing on the moment, but instead dealing with a whole host of things at the same time – with past events, future plans and all the sensations it has to process in the meantime.

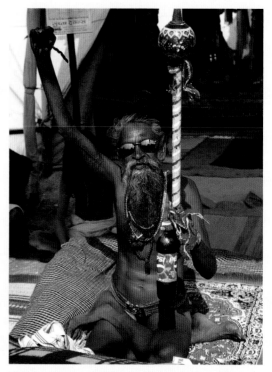

There is no need to go this far to explore the mind: a sadhu or Hindu holy man, who has held up his arm for the last 17 years, in order to repent.

At the same time, the human mind normally interprets everything that is seen, perceived and experienced. It is led by its thought patterns, habits, doctrines, perceptions and conditioning (referred to as *samskara* in Sanskrit), which have been learned during the course of a person's life and have become habit through repetition – irrespective of whether they are good or bad, right or wrong. So it is little wonder that the mind is usually agitated amid all these activities, with the result that human actions are often also blind and unfocused. On the other hand, conscious action requires a clear mind, a mind that has been stilled. Against this background, Patanjali developed the Eight-Limb Path with the aim of stilling the mind.

Aim: a still mind in the here and now

The function of the mind will always be to think and interpret incessantly – after all, that is why it is there. Consequently, the aim of yoga is not to shut out the mind, but rather to enable it to be unaffected by its turnings and instead focus exclusively on a single object or thought. The result of this will be a clear perception that is not clouded by the excessive workings of the mind. If this is achieved, conscious, concentrated action in the here and now – a truly ambitious goal – is made possible. However, the mind permanently places obstacles in the way on the journey towards this goal, and these obstacles are referred to as kleshas (see p.22).

yogascittavrt-tinirodhah

Yoga is when the turnings of the mind cease.
(Yoga Sutra 1.2.)

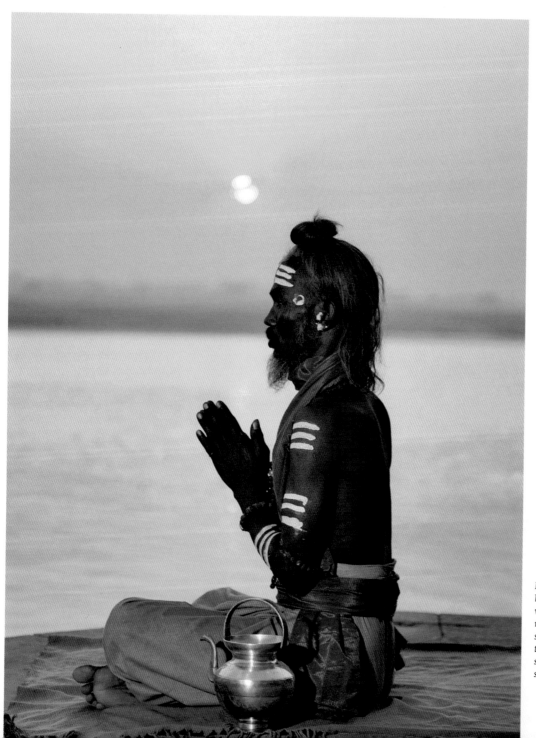

tada drastuh svarupe vasthanam

This produces the ability to go beyond all preconceived ideas and opinions and recognize the truth.
(Yoga Sutra 1.3.)

Holy man meditating on the banks of the Ganges. Even without committing to the religious and in some cases strictly ascetic life followed by the holy men, meditation is still a worthwhile path to self-knowledge.

Kleshas: Afflictions of the mind

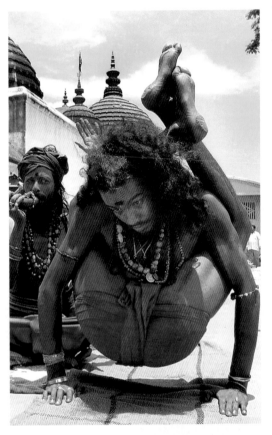

According to Patanjali, a still mind prevents suffering, although it may not appear to be the case.

by previously acquired knowledge, that has been gained through life experiences, wishes and dreams, and particular ideas and expectations – from within oneself and from others. This subjective knowledge is often held to be objective and true, and is used to judge the world. According to Patanjali, this basic deception forms the breeding ground for four further kleshas.

Asmita: The ego – the 'navel' of the world

Asmita refers both to the false estimation of oneself and to an exaggerated egotism. The opinion we have of ourselves may bear little relation to our true self, but it may have been shaped by the perceptions and opinions that others have had of us ever since we were young. This information is instilled into our mind until we come to believe that we really are as others say. This creates feelings of inferiority, or an exaggerated sense of self-worth. According to Patanjali, both of these produce an overstated egotism: our thoughts constantly revolve around ourselves and we see ourselves as the 'navel' of the world.

Patanjali refers to a whole host of obstacles that repeatedly occupy the mind, thereby resulting in suffering. These are divided into five main causes of suffering, or kleshas. Kleshas are fundamental, deep-seated powers – constituting all the human tendencies that hang like a mist over perception and that influence all thoughts and actions. This spiritual resistance prevents us from seeing things clearly and therefore obstructs our path to freedom.

Raga: Craving something again and again

Raga expresses the desire to have needs satisfied and the attachment to pleasurable things – something that can also be expressed in basic greed or addictions. Behind this lie good experiences that a person has had at least once and would like to have again. The craving for happiness is the sole motivation behind actions.

Avidya: Subjective perception

Avidya, ignorance or incorrect knowledge, is the mother of all suffering, because the knowledge through which the world is perceived is invariably subjective rather than objective. Human perception is characterized

Dvesha: Not wanting something (again) under any circumstances

This is used to denote the opposite of raga, namely an exaggerated rejection of things that results from bad experiences or prejudice. Rather than confronting a situation or person

The five kleshas at a glance:
- **Avidya:** ignorance
- **Asmita:** exaggerated egotism
- **Raga:** exaggerated attachment
- **Dvesha:** exaggerated repulsion
- **Abhinivesha:** vague fear (fear of death)

with an open mind, dvesha determines actions, in this case, with stereotypical thinking and negative thoughts.

Abhinivesha: Fear of the unknown

Abhinivesha conceals a vague fear, not necessarily based on experience, but on the assumption that something could go wrong. It is essentially based on the fear of death – fear of complete uncertainty – because nobody knows for sure what happens after death. But because everything is constantly changing and there are no ultimate certainties in life, there are sufficient reasons in everyday life for fear to become all-consuming.

Although fear may be entirely justified and sometimes has a genuinely protective function, the mind is not always able to differentiate between a justified fear and a vague fear of the unknown, and therefore this can have a paralysing effect on it. Consequently, the mind is unable to perceive things accurately, reach decisions or act with clarity. According to Patanjali, the fear klesha has the strongest influence and is the most difficult one to overcome.

Watchfulness and deliberation

The kleshas are not always equally active. Sometimes they work covertly or are barely noticed, while at other times they are highly pronounced and clearly control actions. By being watchful, however, individual kleshas can be tracked down. The important thing is to hesitate, keep automatic impulses in check, break through and then consciously decide how to act. Although Patanjali says that the kleshas can never be completely overcome, the Eight-Limb approach provides methods of significantly reducing their effect on perceptions and on our own actions (see pp.24–31).

This fakir on his bed of nails has clearly managed to overcome his kleshas (c.1930).

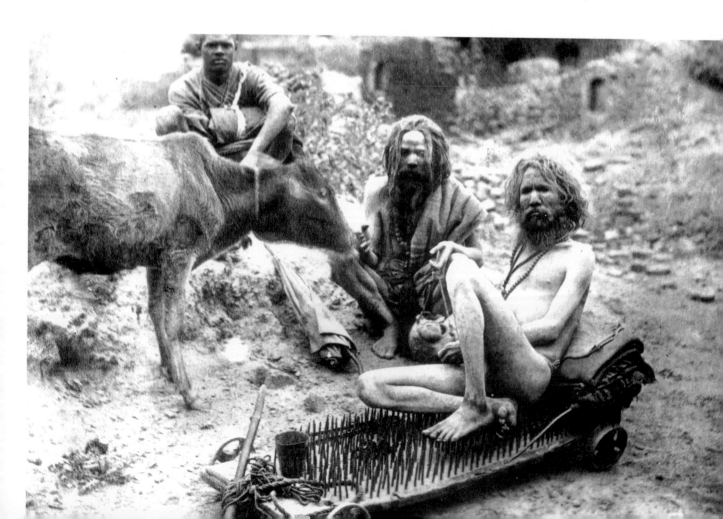

Ashtanga Marga – The Eight-Limb Path
A practical guide to inner freedom

Patanjali wrote that inner freedom and independence could only be achieved by consciously dealing with the afflictions of the mind and reducing their impact on one's own perceptions and actions. The Eight-Limb Path is a sort of self-help guide to overcoming the kleshas; it consists of a series of specific practical approaches and patterns of behaviour that are still very relevant to our lives today.

Yoga is not always an easy or straight road, but it is a worthwhile path to inner freedom.

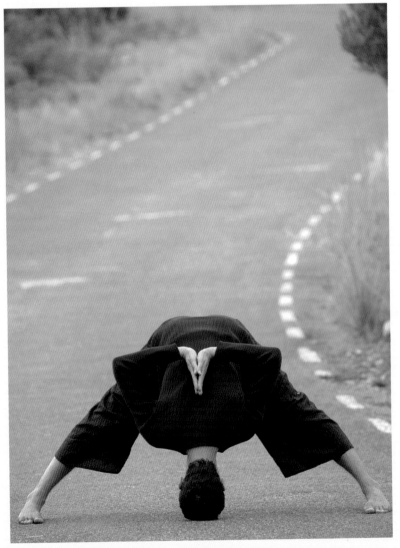

The Eight-Limb Path at a glance

1. *Yamas – dealing with the world around*
2. *Niyamas – dealing with yourself*
3. *Asana – dealing with the body*
4. *Pranayama – dealing with breathing*
5. *Pratyahara – dealing with the senses*

(6–8. *Samyama – dealing with the mind:*)

6. *Dharana – concentration*
7. *Dhyana – meditation*
8. *Samadhi – the Absolute: Inner freedom*

No straight path

Although Patanjali's Ashtanga Marga (from the Sanskrit *ash:* eight; *anga:* limb of a body; and *marga:* path) is referred to as an eight-limb path, it should not be taken to mean that one step necessarily follows the other. Each limb (particularly the first five) provides a doorway in, even though most individuals starting out with yoga do so by practising asanas. Observance of the yamas, or rules of conduct on dealing with the world around us, and the niyamas, or rules on dealing with ourselves, frequently develop through practising asanas. Many people do not practise pranayama or meditation exercises until they have been following their practical training for years. However, the aim of yoga is to consider all limbs equally if possible and to fill them with life on our own path.

Ashtanga Marga is not the same as Ashtanga Yoga

'Ashtanga Marga', the Eight-Limb Path, should not be confused with Ashtanga Yoga, a style of yoga with a fixed series of asana exercises (see p.45).

A worthwhile path

The individual limbs of the Eight-Limb Path can only be developed slowly – something known by the author of the Yoga Sutras. Reaching the point of perfect freedom is more than difficult (and this is immediately evident to anyone who has tried it). It must be viewed as an ongoing process of continuing development, rather than a quick route to enlightenment. But even if you never manage to get rid of your kleshas and their samskaras completely, it is a truly worthwhile path to take. With continuous practice and an open heart and mind (which is where Patanjali believed human self-knowledge is hidden), it is possible to gradually free yourself from limiting habits or patterns of behaviour that may be creating obstructions and to escape from the opinions and expectations of others. The Eight-Limb Path at least teaches you to recognize these more readily and to deal with them more consciously. And who knows, perhaps you will achieve that vast inner freedom one day after all!

Practise, practise – and practise some more

Reducing the effect of the kleshas and clearing the mind requires continual practice and will not happen overnight. Everyone should find their level and sustain it over a prolonged period. The other important thing is to make sure that you let go of everything else (which in many cases is outside your own power anyway) and that means taking things as they come. The basic belief that you are on the right path helps in both cases.

trayamanta-
rangam pur-
vebhyah

Compared with the first limbs of the path, the last three mentioned are difficult.
(Yoga Sutra 3.7.)

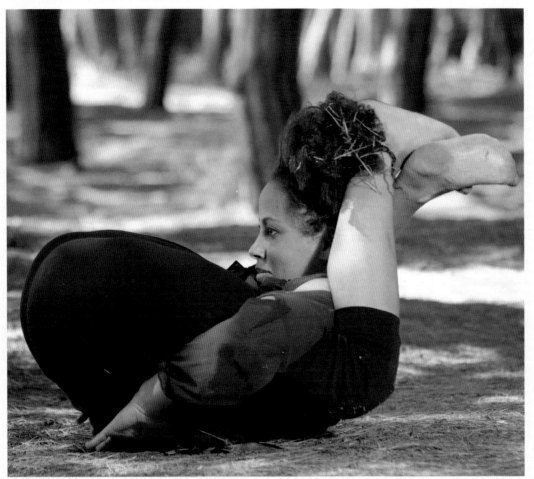

abhyasavai-
ragyabhyam
tannirodhah

Through practice and the ability to let go, the mind can achieve and maintain the state of yoga.
(Yoga Sutra 1.12.)

Being able to execute this asana, called Yoga Nidrasana (yoga sleep pose), and find it relaxing at the same time requires a great deal of practice and a highly developed ability to let go and attain great stillness of mind.

The Eight-Limb Path – 1st limb:
Dealing with the world around

ahimsasatya-
steyabrahma-
caryaaparigrha
yamah

Non-violence,
truthfulness, non-
stealing, moderation
and non-covetousness
are the outward
disciplines.
(Yoga Sutra 2.30.)

1st limb: The yamas

The yamas lay down five moral principles that
govern the way you treat others and the world
around you.

Ahimsa: Non-violence

Ahimsa goes far beyond purely physical non-
violence; it involves recognizing not only
destructive deeds, but words and thoughts
too, and banishing them from your own life
wherever possible. This includes treating the
environment, other living beings and, not
least, yourself with awareness and respect. It
is essential to develop a profound sensitivity
towards all living beings and to calculate in
each situation the conduct that will cause
least damage.

Satya: Truthfulness

Satya not only deals with unconditional
honesty, but also genuine conduct. It involves
not saying anything that is untrue, not
even through misplaced thoughtfulness. In
addition, satya means not only thinking about
what is said, but also *how* it is said and what
consequences the truth will hold. The aim is
to formulate the truth in the best possible way,
without harming anyone, either intentionally
or unintentionally.

Asteya: Non-stealing

Asteya includes not taking what is not yours –
and no distinction is made between material
goods, actions or thoughts. Claiming the
credit for something undeservedly, stealing
someone else's ideas or abusing another's
trust is just as much a violation of asteya
in this sense as stealing the silver. The property
of others must always be respected.

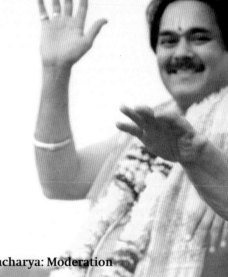

Brahmacharya: Moderation

Brahmacharya involves moderation in all
areas of life and concentrating on the divine.
All excess, dependences and extremes can
lead to thoughts and actions being completely
dictated by these. It is precisely this that
brahmacharya can be used to prevent. This
concept does not require complete abstinence
(either from stimulants or regular habits),
but expects you to find the right balance, not
to surrender yourself to your passions, and
thereby to remain independent.

Brahmacharya was originally taken to mean
celibacy and asceticism, based on the thinking
that anything not directed at the essential
(that being the search for truth) is simply a
waste of energy.

Aparigraha: Non-covetousness

The concept of aparigraha is similar to that of
asteya, except that it focuses more on the inner
attitude of moderation. It involves conscious
reflection on what and how much a person
actually needs of something (not only food, space,
etc., but also fame or acknowledgement); this may
differ greatly from one individual to the next.
The crucial point about aparigraha is to become
free of expectations and the desire to possess.

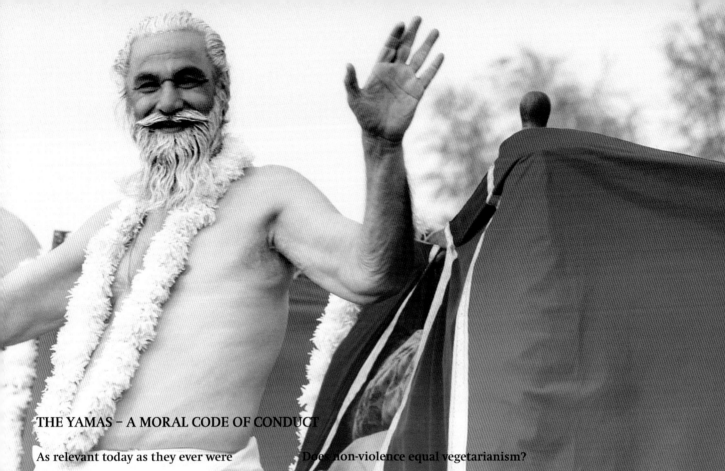

THE YAMAS – A MORAL CODE OF CONDUCT

As relevant today as they ever were

The yamas represent a moral code of conduct – in some respects Patanjali can be regarded as being one of the earliest environmentalists. Climate change, dwindling resources, increasing health problems (both physical and psychological) among his contemporaries and the growing propensity for violence all highlight how relevant the morality of yoga is today.

Finding personal well-being through the yamas

Observing the yamas may lead to harmony within yourself and with your surroundings. The less the mind identifies with life's stresses, the stiller it becomes. The more your views are shaped by the yamas, the greater the atmosphere of peace generated around you. The more positive a person is in their outlook, the more positive the return. And the more liberated a person is from covetousness and dependences, the greater the serenity felt within. In turn, the greater the inner serenity, the simpler your own life appears and the easier it becomes to handle what life throws at you.

Does non-violence equal vegetarianism?

Many yogis today refer to the subject of vegetarianism in connection with ahimsa. For these practitioners, being a vegetarian is a matter of course, but you will find that opinions on whether or not it is essential vary greatly. Nevertheless, anyone who practises yoga will in time develop a greater awareness and also a deeper respect for all living beings, so that they will listen more and more to their own physical feelings, without having to follow dogma.

Everyday living – a huge challenge

Abiding by the yamas is a huge challenge in everyday life. Each day the yoga student will be confronted on numerous occasions with the question of how far the yamas can be observed. Ultimately, there are very few people who are saintly or even aspire to be. Consequently, you have to give yourself some consideration too and be relaxed and good-humoured in your progression, but also notice setbacks in your observance of the yamas and view this path as an ongoing process.

The Eight-Limb Path – 2nd limb:
Dealing with yourself

*The niyama saucha (purity)
is not only a question of
outer cleanliness, but also an
attitude within.*

2nd limb: The niyamas

The niyamas are the five observances, or rules of conduct, by which we should live our lives. These include:

Saucha: Purity

At a physical level, saucha not only means regular daily hygiene, but also maintaining an awareness of diet and keeping the body pure by continually practising asanas. The yogi's immediate environment – his clothing or home, for example – is also affected by this. At a spiritual level, saucha means keeping thoughts pure and being guided by consideration.

Santosha: Contentment

Santosha refers to what we have and what we are content to be – whether on a material, physical or intellectual level. This presupposes acceptance of ourselves and our personal circumstances. However, santosha does not mean we should stop developing and learning, but rather that inner contentment should not be dependent on external factors.

Tapas: Self-discipline

Self-discipline arises from a 'burning desire' (from the Sanskrit *tapah*, meaning 'heat') and an inner need. This burning desire is the fuel that enables us to tackle challenges with persistence and stamina, in order to reach self-awareness.

Svadhyaya: Self-study, self-reflection

Svadhyaya traditionally means studying the sacred texts (Patanjali's Yoga Sutras or the Bhagavad Gita, for example) as a means of self-discovery. However, it also denotes the ability to observe, analyse and reflect on ourselves and our behaviour. What this means

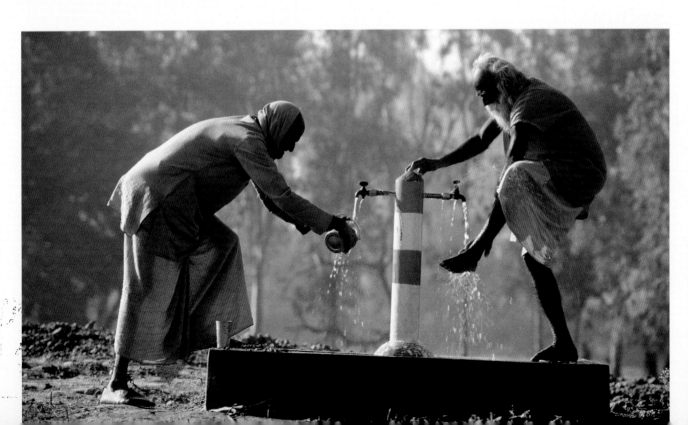

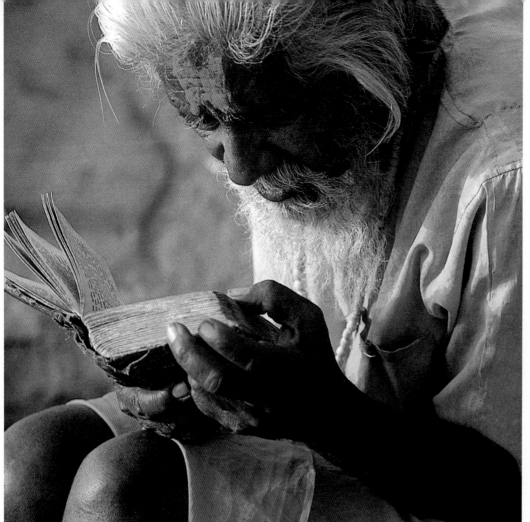

The niyama svadhyaya traditionally includes self-study and the reading of the sacred texts.

Yoga practice must incorporate three qualities: discipline, self-study and acceptance of our own limits.
(Yoga Sutra 2.1.)

is that we should continually be aware of what influences our behaviour, which stimulus-response patterns we may be governed by and what the causes of these are.

Ishvarapranidhana: Faith in a higher force

The last niyama requires us to acknowledge our own boundaries and to accept that many things are not within our power to change. Whether this acceptance or 'letting go' takes the form of devotion to a divinity or higher force or simply a basic belief in life itself is left up to each individual.

Incorporating the niyamas in our everyday lives

However enlightening the niyamas may seem as a guide to handling ourselves, they can sometimes also appear impossible to enforce in everyday life. Keeping the body clean still appears simple, but every thought too? This is more difficult. Contentment is also constantly being tested in the face of innumerable everyday temptations. 'Burning desires' and discipline are all too often put in check by a sudden, inexplicable inertia. Self-reflection can be tiresome and how often would we prefer not to look into our own deep abysses? On the other hand, it seems easy to identify our own limits, although this does stop us from wrestling with them. Only one thing helps: carrying on, not asking too much of ourselves, taking small steps and not allowing ourselves to be thrown by setbacks.

Patanjali's yoga kriyas more or less summarize the Eight-Limb Path: the three forms of conduct comprising discipline, self-study and acceptance of ourselves are highlighted as particularly effective by Patanjali.

The Eight-Limb Path – 3rd–8th limb:
Dealing with the body, breathing, the senses and the mind

sthirasukhama-
sanam

Asanas should combine
the qualities of stability
and effortlessness in
equal measure.
(Yoga Sutra 2.46.)

tato dvan-
dvanabhigatahj

A person who practises
asanas correctly cannot
be unsettled by extreme
external influences.
(Yoga Sutra 2.48.)

tatah ksi-
yate prakasa-
varanam

Practising pranayama
regularly reduces the
obstructions that prevent
clear perception.
(Yoga Sutra 2.52.)

3rd limb: Asana

Nowadays, performing the physical postures, or asanas, generally constitutes most of yoga practice. Patanjali's Yoga Sutras only mention sitting (from the Sanskrit *asana*, meaning 'to sit' or 'to stay'). However, the qualities required here can be transferred to all asanas developed later.

Finding harmony in conflict

Patanjali's Yoga Sutras mention two qualities that the asanas should combine: stability and effortlessness. When the body is firmly focused on the asana it becomes grounded, producing stability. An energetic effortlessness is simultaneously achieved by approaching the limit of our own potential, but never crossing it, so that the asana can be held with a degree of effortlessness and pleasure. There is more on the subject of stability and effortlessness in the chapters on the asanas.

4th limb: Pranayama

Pranayama denotes a conscious control of energy, in other words, controlling and expanding the breathing. By practising controlled breathing techniques, the body and mind are relaxed and obstacles are removed, so that there is a better energy flow. There is more on this in the pranayama chapter (see pp.216–23).

5th limb: Pratyahara

Pratyahara denotes the withdrawal of the senses. These are like the open doors of the mind that are sought out by everything that wants to pass through the doors and reach the mind. On the one hand, this is indispensable to life, because the senses create the contact with the outside world. On the other hand, there is a constant risk of being bombarded by stimuli and being distracted from concentrating on one task. Pratyahara teaches us to close the doors to the senses, so that the mind is still aware of external stimuli but no longer responds to them.

6th–8th limbs: Samyama

Samyama covers the last three limbs of the path, which deal exclusively with the mind. While the other five limbs of the yoga practice path serve to still the mind and prepare it for the path to inner freedom, samyama goes right to the core of self-knowledge.

6th limb: Dharana

Dharana denotes the ability to focus our entire concentration on an object, an action, a question or consideration and keep it there. It is only this sort of concentration that makes a deeper penetration and understanding of the object of concentration possible.

7th limb: Dhyana

In meditation there is a sort of interaction with the object of concentration. During meditation, the subjective notions of knowledge, thought patterns, doctrines, expectations and emotions are left behind and things are intuitively seen as they actually are. We view as an observer what was previously chosen as an object of meditation. The neutral observer accepts everything they see, without evaluating or assessing it, without intervening or seeking to change anything. There is more on this in the chapter on meditation (see p.224).

8th limb: Samadhi

At the end of the path lies the Absolute, which is the state of inner freedom. Patanjali's Yoga Sutras describe this as a complete feeling of oneness with the object of meditation. In this state feelings of one's own identity are lost. There are countless other ways of describing samadhi: knowledge of the true self, or enlightenment, or feeling at one with the world as a whole or with something divine. Inner happiness is a state of absolute freedom that is independent of outside circumstances.

Lotus blossom is a symbol of purity in Hinduism and Buddhism. Yogis also see it as the symbol of samadhi – the Absolute.

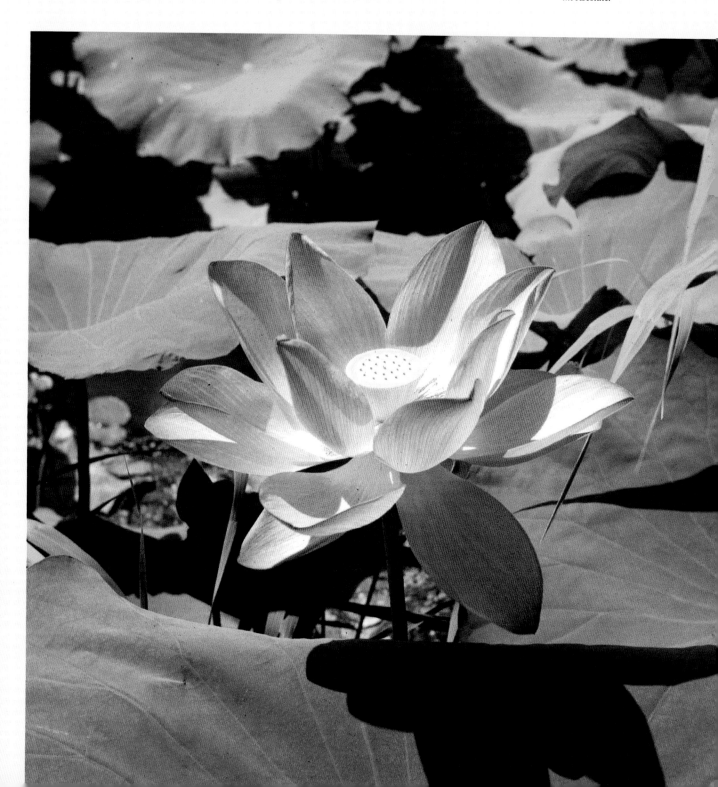

HATHA YOGA

The body as a tool

Hatha Yoga Pradipika
ha: sun; *tha:* moon; *yoga:*
to unify; *Pradipika:* torch
(light on)

Rooted in the Tantric movement (see box, p.33), whose proponents in the early 6th century developed the idea that everything that exists – including the body – is an expression of the divine, Hatha Yoga emerged some time around the 9th century AD. Hatha Yoga is a form of yoga that focuses on the body. The aim of this is still fundamental knowledge, but the route taken is not through meditation, but physical exercises.

Hatha Yoga Pradipika was a guide to a series of practical exercises, which are still relevant today, albeit in slightly modified form, and practised by the majority of yogis. Hatha Yoga therefore became the generic term for all body-based styles of yoga and stands for the channelling of energies within the body.

Male and female energy

In Hatha Yoga, the path to knowledge begins not with meditation, but physical exercises.

Male energy is symbolized by the sun (*ha* in Sanskrit) and is associated with warmth, motivation, drive, resolve, activity and the extrovert side of the individual, emphasizing understanding. Female energy is depicted by the moon (*tha* in Sanskrit) and is associated with coolness, passivity, imagination and the emotional, loving, intuitive side of the individual. Although the world is made up of dualisms, everything that at first seems opposing emerges in Hatha Yoga as two sides of the same coin that belong together. Hatha Yoga therefore aims to unify these two sides and bring them into harmony.

The energetic body

Hatha Yoga goes beyond the purely anatomical structure in its contemplation of the body and considers that not only diet, but also all emotions, injuries and thoughts are stored in the body and lead to tension and the obstruction of energy. These obstructions have to be unblocked so that the life force can flow freely. For this reason, Hatha yogis place greatest emphasis on strengthening their own bodies during their yoga practice.

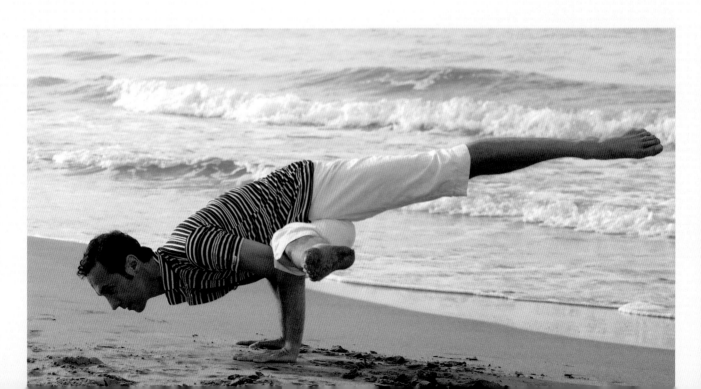

Structure of the energetic body

The energetic body is made up of prana (the life force), koshas (the sheaths of the body), nadis (the energy channels), which transport prana through the body, and chakras, the energy centres and main junctions of the nadis (see pp.34–7). The energetic body cannot be demonstrated by conventional medicine. As a result, many people (particularly in the West) find it difficult to begin to imagine the existence of the energetic body. In order to work with the body's energy, for most people it is enough to imagine and visualize images connected to the energetic body, so that they can concentrate on given points in the body and channel energy there.

Tantrism

Tantrism is a religious movement that has had a significant influence on Hinduism and Buddhism since the 5th century. The Tantric texts (tantras) describe the differences between the macrocosm and microcosm, the universal and the individual soul, man and woman (not seen as a genuine duality, and their 'redemption' as their reunification in the originally undivided one).

Tantrism is readily associated with sexual rites, particularly in the West. In actual fact, Tantrics regard the body as holy. But the physical rituals and practices are used spiritually, to unify the cosmic consciousness (Shiva) and cosmic energy (Shakti) within the body and thereby attain the highest level of happiness. The body acts as a bridge to unify Purusha and Prakriti (see p.18).

Although this position from the Kama Sutra is clearly reminiscent of yogic asanas and Tantrism is readily associated with sexual rites, the movement is primarily concerned with the spiritual union of male and female energy.

The anatomy of Hatha Yoga
Koshas, prana and nadis

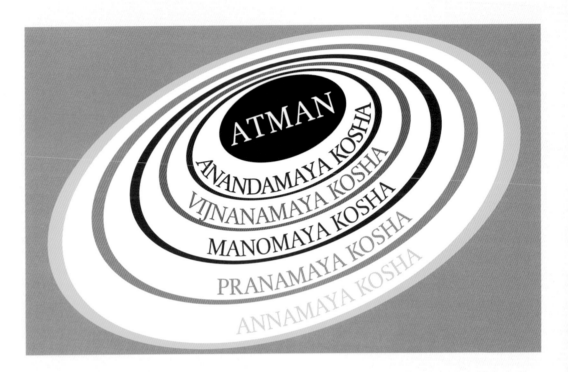

Diagram of the koshas –
the body's five sheaths.

Koshas:
The five sheaths, or levels, of the body

Hatha Yoga is based on five sheaths, or levels, of the body. These are not separate from one another, but progress from the dense to the subtle levels – from the outside in. This is one of the oldest images of the body, which was around at the time of the Upanishads.

Annamaya kosha: The physical body

This is the only tangible sheath – made up of the five elements. It is earth, fire, water, air and space – and constitutes the physical body.

Pranamaya kosha: The energetic body

This refers to the body's vital level, which supplies both the physical and spiritual body with energy. In terms of dense matter, this sheath consists of the circulatory, respiratory and metabolic systems; at the subtle level, this refers to all energy channels that transport prana through the body. Pranamaya kosha represents the bridge between the body and the spirit. Consequently, Hatha Yoga exercises are added at this level to influence the spirit and emotional condition of the practitioner.

Manomaya kosha: The information body

This sheath is the instrument that gathers information on the sensations and is at the same time home to all wishes, needs, feelings, fears and memories. At this sheath, or level, unconscious messages are constantly transmitted back and forth between the sheaths of the body.

Vijnanamaya kosha: The wisdom body

This level is the place of intelligence that is capable of observing and discriminating, analysing, reflecting and interpreting information that is supplied to the manomaya kosha. Ideally, decisions are made at this level of consciousness, which lead to conscious action.

Anandamaya kosha: The bliss body

At the centre of the koshas is bliss. This level of consciousness, which conceals the essence of the individual soul (Atman), is achieved by those who have come to terms with themselves and the world and who are unaffected by Karma, samskaras or kleshas.

Prana: The life force

Prana is the life force circulating in the body. By using various breathing techniques combined with physical practice, the Hatha yogi tries to locate resistance in the body. Using individual exercises, he channels energy right to these points to remove blockages. In so doing, he turns on the light, figuratively speaking, in order to see more and achieve a higher spiritual level.

Nadis: The body's energy channels

Nadis refer to the energy channels that transport life force (prana) within the body. Tradition has it that there are 72,000 nadis, which the rishis (Indian sages) have found through deep meditation. The three most important nadis are sushumna, ida and pingala.

Sushumna This starts at the tailbone and runs through the spine along the chakras to the middle of the back of the head. It is not normally active and only has a small energy flow, because it is blocked by resistance in the body and spirit.

Ida and pingala Both begin at the base of the spine, meander around the spine and cross six times below the chakras up to the nostrils. Ida ends on the left and is associated with female energy; pingala ends on the right and is associated with male energy. Ida and pingala connect the left and right halves of the body.

Activating sushumna When sushumna is not active, energy flows alternately through the two nadis (at roughly 60–90 minute intervals). Normally, the energy flow is not therefore

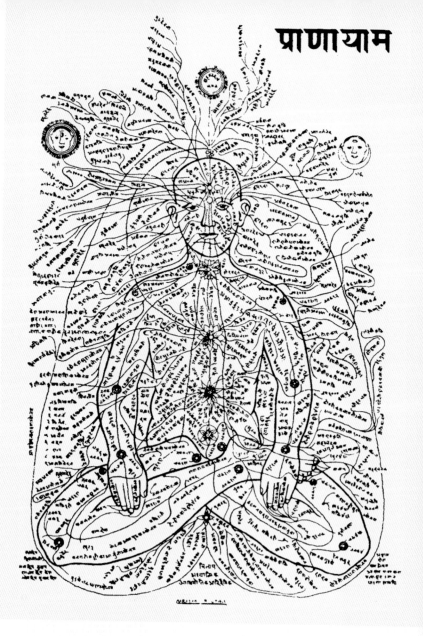

प्राणायाम

balanced. The Hatha yogi seeks to balance ida and pingala, because only then is sushumna unblocked and activated. When energy is able to flow through sushumna, the chakras are activated. When there are no blocks there and the energy flow is strong enough, energy shoots straight into the last chakra (in the crown of the head), where universal consciousness is able to combine with individual consciousness.

Diagram of the nadis in Sanskrit: tradition has it that 72,000 energy channels run through the human body.

The anatomy of Hatha Yoga
Chakras and kundalini

Chakras: The body's energy centres

Chakras denote the energy centres of the body (seven in total), which run like a string of pearls from the base of the spine to the crown of the head. The word 'chakra' translates as 'wheel', so each chakra can be visualized as a sort of fly-wheel that transports energy from one level to the next. Each of the chakras has its own distinct characteristics and corresponds to a unique aspect of our being. Chakras can be open or closed and a state of equilibrium is only achieved when all chakras are open and energy can flow freely from bottom to top. However, physical and spiritual obstructions, which can manifest themselves in any of the chakras, mean that this is not always possible. Hatha Yoga techniques help to overcome these obstructions.

The seven chakras, or energy centres, run along the spinal column.

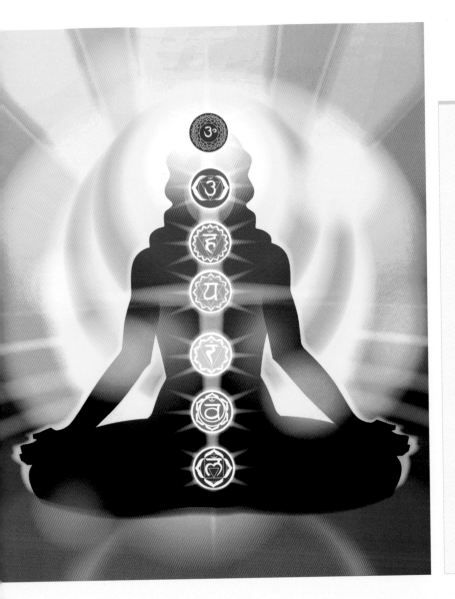

Bringing kundalini, the snake, to life

According to tradition, kundalini (from the Sanskrit for 'snake') lies coiled at the base of the sushumna, blocking its energy flow. A balanced energy flow in the other two main nadis (see p.35) and active chakras arouses kundalini, uncoils it and leaves the way free for the cosmic energy (shakti), which is finally able to ascend the sushumna and be unified with the cosmic consciousness (Shiva). Shakti feels infinite delight and deep joy at finally being where she is at home. Based on this mythological image, Hatha Yoga is frequently also called Kundalini Yoga. Many schools of yoga devote themselves specifically to kundalini, using exercises to prepare the body for the ascending energy. The aim is to purify the chakras, so that kundalini can ascend unobstructed. In modern-day yoga, kundalini is also compared to inner temptation, which must be overcome in practice by constantly developing greater resistance or building bigger energy blocks and confronting it.

Kundalini describes the coiled serpent. Those who succeed in mobilizing this force will without the slightest doubt be liberated.
(Hatha Yoga Pradipika III, 108)

Finding self-knowledge by concentrating on the chakras

By concentrating on the chakras during his exercise techniques, the Hatha yogi tries to gain self-knowledge to discover where negative traits have led to 'energy blocks' and to develop protective mechanisms. As with any other type of yoga, the Hatha Yoga path seeks liberation from these blockages and the attainment of a holistic consciousness of the unit.

In practice, this involves using the individual elements assigned to the chakras (see table below), in order to strengthen concentration on the chakras. This means, for example, that colours are visualized or mantras sung, in order to set the chakras in motion, which can be imagined as wheels.

The seven chakras at a glance

Each chakra is assigned certain elements, which can be included when concentrating on the energy centres.

Chakra	Assignment	Associated with...
1. Muladhara chakra 'Root support' Base chakra Base of the spine chakra	Position: Pelvic floor Element: Earth Sense: Smell Colour: Red Mantra: Lam	...the ability to feel grounded in life. Key words: stability, family, childhood, basic trust, base, society, conditioning, fear of existence
2. Svadhisthana chakra 'Place of the self' Sacral chakra	Position: Abdomen Element: Water Sense: Taste Colour: Orange Mantra: Vam	...what constitutes our own identity. Key words: gender, sexuality, creativity, dualism, propagation
3. Manipura chakra 'Town of jewels' Solar plexus chakra Navel chakra	Position: Upper abdomen Element: Fire Sense: Sight Colour: Yellow Mantra: Ram	...what constitutes our own self. Key words: self-consciousness, self-worth, self-confidence, drive, development, power
4. Anahata chakra 'Unstruck (mystical) note' Heart chakra	Position: Heart Element: Air Sense: Touch Colour: Green Mantra: Yam	....all emotional subjects. Key words: love, sympathy, sadness, pain, devotion, rage, hatred, joy
5. Vishuddha chakra 'The loud, pure' Neck chakra Throat chakra	Position: Neck Element: Ether Sense: Hearing Colour: Blue Mantra: Ham	...attentive manipulation and interpretation of the senses. Key words: authenticity, inner attitude, will, honesty, communication, expression of energies
6. Ajna chakra 'Place of the command' Brow chakra 'Third eye' chakra	Position: Forehead Element: Mental powers (fine) Sense: Balance Colour: Dark blue or indigo Mantra: Om	...the ability to know ourselves, to see life and ourselves as they really are. Key words: brain functions, understanding, logic, analysis, reflection, contemplation, intuition, self-awareness
7. Sahasrara chakra 'Thousand-petalled lotus' Head chakra Crown of the head chakra	Position: Top of the head Element: None assigned Sense: None assigned Colour: Purple Mantra: Inner sound	...the ability to be in harmony with ourselves and all around us. Key words: solidarity, true seeing, inner and outer unity, true nature, true self, samadhi, enlightenment, freedom, bliss, the Absolute, connection to God or a higher energy

Hatha Yoga exercise techniques

Asana

Asana practice – performing the physical postures – is a central feature of Hatha Yoga. The asanas described in the Hatha Yoga Pradipika focus on the spine and are intended to stimulate and guide the central energy. Over the centuries, a whole host of asanas has developed that also concentrate entirely on the spine. For more information about asanas see pp.50–53 and pp.234–5.

You need a good teacher and lots of practice to learn nauli, the cleansing of the digestive organs. The digestive organs are turned in the abdomen as if in a spin-dryer.

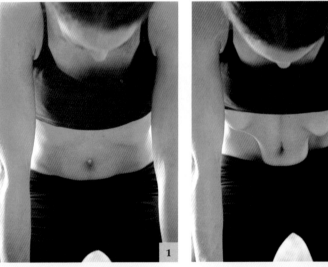

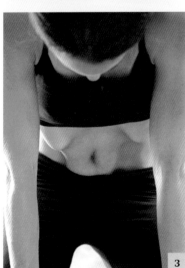

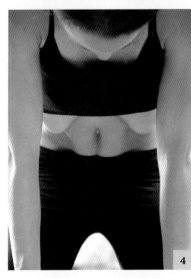

Balanced diet

The Hatha Yoga Pradipika includes diet recommendations that are still relevant today. Food should be fresh, easy to digest, taken in moderation and varied – in other words, a mixed, balanced diet, which should also be enjoyable and eaten in peace.

There is no specific ban on eating meat or fish, although it is pointed out that these are unsuitable for yogis. However, there is no indication of whether this recommendation stems back to ahimsa (non-violence, see p.26) or is purely a reflection on meat being harder to digest than vegetables.

Shat Karma Kriya: Cleansing rituals

The cleansing rituals are practised to purify the physical body and the energy channels, or nadis. In some cases, they are completely alien to Western students and should only be tried in a limited number of cases. Anyone wishing to learn these should be guided by a teacher who has a good command of the techniques.

Dhauti: inner cleansing of the chest, stomach and intestine
Basti/Vasti: external cleansing of the excretory organs
Neti: cleansing of the respiratory organs
Trataka: cleansing of the eyes
Nauli: cleansing of the digestive organs
Kapalabhati: cleansing of the inner head space and lungs

Bandhas: The body's locks

Bandhas are the body's locks (*bandha* meaning 'lock' or 'seal' in Sanskrit), enabling energy to be kept in the body and better regulated and controlled. In short, they optimize the energy flow. For more on how the bandhas are used in practice, see p.52.

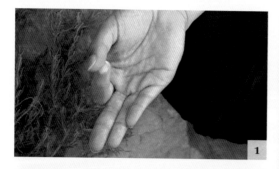

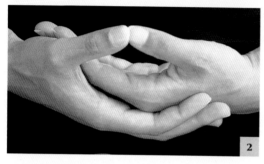

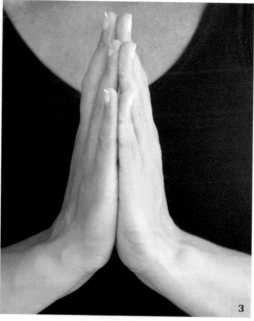

Taken from the vast array of mudras, here is a small selection of the most important ones.

1. Jnana mudra: The unification of the individual self (index finger) with the cosmos (thumb).

2. Dhyana mudra: The meditation gesture. It transforms each attachment to clear perception.

3. Anjali mudra: This mudra means offering or devotion. It is frequently associated with the word 'Namaste', which translates as 'The divinity in me bows to the divinity in you'.

Mudras: The body's seals

Mudras are gestures involving the hands that concentrate the energy flow. They help the energy within the body to be consciously experienced and guided. The different mudras also each have a symbolic significance.

Pranayama and meditation

The explanations of these subjects in Hatha Yoga do not differ significantly from Patanjali's Eight-Limb Path – see p.28 and the chapters on pranayama (pp.216–23) and meditation (pp.224–31).

Listening to the inner sound

This refers to the chanting of 'OM' (see right), which can be sung in many different variants. It is often started three times in succession in order to collect oneself. The continuous chanting of OM is also widespread. It begins softly, becoming louder and then quieter again, until it is completely silent. This is followed by concentration on the inner sound, an inner vibration that cleanses the energy paths and removes any blockages. The aim is to hear *anahata nadam*, the sound of stillness.

The aim: Samadhi

As in Patanjali's Eight-Limb Path, samadhi, or inner freedom, is the aim of Hatha Yoga exercises (see p.28). The Hatha Yoga Pradipika describes various phenomena that occur when the yogi is liberated. He is '... free from all thoughts ... can transcend time ... is unaware of smells, tastes, touch, noise or even himself or others ... is neither awake nor asleep, he ... is unaware of heat or cold, luck or misfortune ... is apparently sleeping while awake, without breathing in or out ... he cannot be injured by any weapon or power in this world'.

The path is the goal

This explanation may be sufficient to illustrate that the path of Hatha Yoga, in a similar way to Patanjali's Eight-Limb Path, is not necessarily suitable for those lacking patience. The path to attaining the state of samadhi is a difficult one, but every single step taken towards it makes us less dependent on external influences and helps us develop an ever-greater inner calm in how we deal with the world in all its guises.

The holy mantra OM

The syllable OM is the most sacred mantra and is sung by yogis, Hindus and Buddhists alike. OM is the universal primeval sound. In Sanskrit, OM is made up of the syllables 'A', 'U' and 'M', which are combined to produce 'O' and the nasal sound 'M'. Numerous meanings are given to these three letters – although they are usually associated with the beginning, the middle and the end – and the syllable OM is thereby understood to depict reality in its entirety.

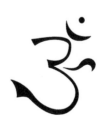

At a glance:

THE MAIN PATHS OF HISTORICAL YOGA

Satsang (from the Sanskrit *satya*, 'truth', and *anga*, 'limb'): a community of individuals seeking the truth. It is important to surround yourself with people who do good and who are true and genuine.

The history of yoga is essentially associated with five main paths, which are often combined together in today's practice, since they are in no way at odds and in many cases complement one another.

Yoga paths in the Bhagavad Gita

There are three yoga paths identified in the Bhagavad Gita that have had a sustained influence on the practice of yoga to date:

1. Bhakti Yoga: The path of devotion leads to something higher, something life-determining, to freedom. Associated with this is acceptance of our own fate and the belief that all experiences are guided by a higher power and are for our own good. This path focuses on love, devotion and sympathy. One of the methods that supports the Bhakti Yoga path is chanting or the singing of devotional prayers and songs of praise to God, with which Bhakti Yoga expresses its devotion to a higher power.

2. Karma Yoga: The path of conscious action is based on the principle of acting consciously and selflessly, irrespective of inclination and preference. The aim is to avoid or at least mitigate suffering, as far as possible. In Karma Yoga, individuals are not only responsible for each of their actions – whether in thought, word or deed – but also for the consequences of these. The Dharma, or duty in life, must be adhered to – irrespective of the reward.

3. Jnana Yoga: The path of wisdom is trodden with the help of knowledge, understanding, intellect and the ability to discriminate. The Jnana yogi achieves self-awareness firstly through the spiritual search for truth, by studying the old texts and recognizing the structure of the mind through self-reflection; secondly, meditation enables him to penetrate beyond the intellect, thereby achieving further intuitive knowledge. A Jnana yogi assumes that learning is an ongoing process in which anything can be the teacher: the ancient texts, gurus (teachers) and satsangs (associations of truth-seekers), as well as everyday life.

Raja Yoga

This movement, also known as the royal path, is based on the Yoga Sutras of Patanjali (see pp.20–31). The Raja yogi follows the Eight-Limb Path of Patanjali, giving particular significance to the last three limbs. His spirit, body and breath are the tools he needs to achieve self-awareness.

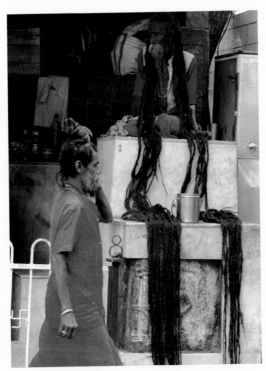

No matter which yoga path is followed, it will require a great deal of patience.

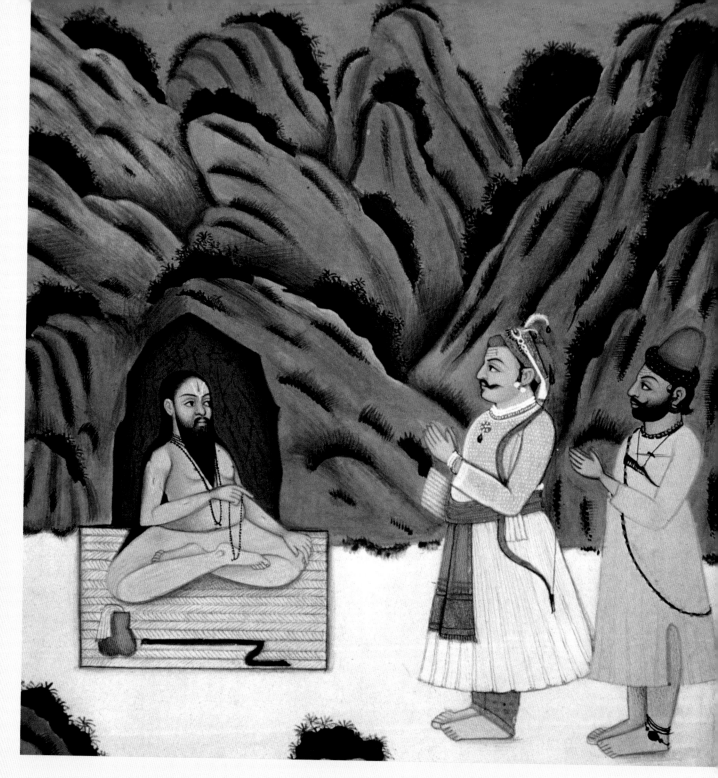

Hatha Yoga

The path of physicality emerged under the influence of Tantrism (see box, p.33) and led firstly to an encounter with the Absolute, not only through meditation and self-awareness, but increasingly through physical exercises.

These are still practised by most yogis today – albeit in modified form. In Hatha Yoga, everything centres on energy work aimed at guiding the energy flow. The fundamental text for this movement is the Hatha Yoga Pradipika (see pp.32–9).

In early times, wise yogis often withdrew from everyday life, opting for an ascetic existence. Some yogis continue this tradition today, although most yoga practitioners integrate their path into their daily routine.

MODERN YOGA

Yoga goes West

Hatha Yoga remained very popular in India well into the 16th century. However, the development of a fundamentalist tendency in Hinduism led to members of the lower castes as well as women being excluded from the yoga exercise path. This resulted in the path of yoga disappearing almost completely from

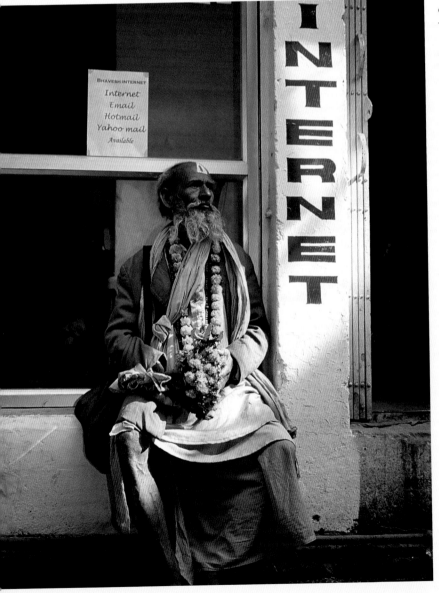

A Sadhu or Hindu holy man sitting outside an Internet cafe in Varanasi. Yoga became part of the modern world long ago.

Indian life. Nevertheless, the knowledge of yoga was retained for centuries and underwent a renaissance in the second half of the 19th century that was felt far beyond India. This was begun primarily by new religious movements that reinvigorated the old yoga practices. One of those to rediscover yoga was the Indian philosopher Sri Aurobindo Ghose (1872–1950), who with his concept of 'integral yoga' tried to create a connection between all religions that was free from dogma.

First steps in the West

Swami Vivekananda (1863–1902), one of the founders of new Hinduism, devoted his life to the goal of introducing the West to the Vedic texts. The year 1893, when Vivekananda made a speech to the Parliament of the World's Religions in Chicago, can be regarded as the year in which yoga was born in the West. It was here that Vivekananda introduced for the first time a large Western audience to the yoga practices developed over thousands of years by the rishis (Indian sages) in their search for spiritual happiness. This marked the beginning of yoga's unstoppable movement from East to West.

The modernizers of ancient traditions

Among many other yogis, two Indians in particular created yoga as it is known today all over the world: Swami Sivananda Saraswati and Tirumalai Krishnamacharya.

Swami Sivananda Saraswati (1887–1963) developed a style of yoga that combined Karma, Jnana, Bhakti and Raja Yoga (see p.40). According to Sivananda, this combination of styles can be used to overcome all life's challenges. Gentle asana practice, to keep the body healthy, is just as much a part of this as meditation for stilling the mind.

Tirumalai Krishnamacharya (1888–1989) almost uniquely symbolized the body-based yoga that is taught and practised in numerous different styles in the West today. He began learning yoga and Sanskrit as a child, and went on to study logic, grammar and philosophy before finally training in Ayurvedic medicine. His knowledge of yoga was developed by spending seven years in the Himalayas with his teacher, Ramamohan Brahmachari.

In accordance with his teacher's wishes, Krishnamacharya chose not to become a scholar and instead went on to teach yoga. He founded the Mysore school, where he gradually began teaching women and taking on pupils from the West. His most famous pupils included B.K.S. Iyengar, Patthabi Jois and T.K.V. Desikachar (see p.45). Krishnamacharya regularly toured India to bring yoga back to the people. He was regarded as the undisputed godfather of modern-day Hatha Yoga and all body-based styles developed subsequently have their roots in Krishnamacharya's yoga.

Krishnamacharya placed the benefits of the physical practice at the centre of his teachings, alongside the spiritual practice. He did not teach a general form of yoga for the masses, but familiarized each of his pupils with yoga in an individual way. Each of his pupils received their own personal exercise programme. For example, he would provide young people with a series of demanding exercise sequences that built on one another, and constantly presented practitioners with a fresh challenge. In order to improve his pupils' concentration, he combined their asanas with breathing exercises and allowed the sequences of one asana to flow into the next (see Vinyasa Yoga, p.47). In this way, he prepared his students for a spiritual development, which, despite the focus on asana practice, was for Krishnamacharya the aim of yoga. For the sick, on the other hand, he set targeted asana and breathing exercises combined with Ayurvedic healing treatments, seeing illness as an obstacle on the path to spiritual development that had to be alleviated and removed.

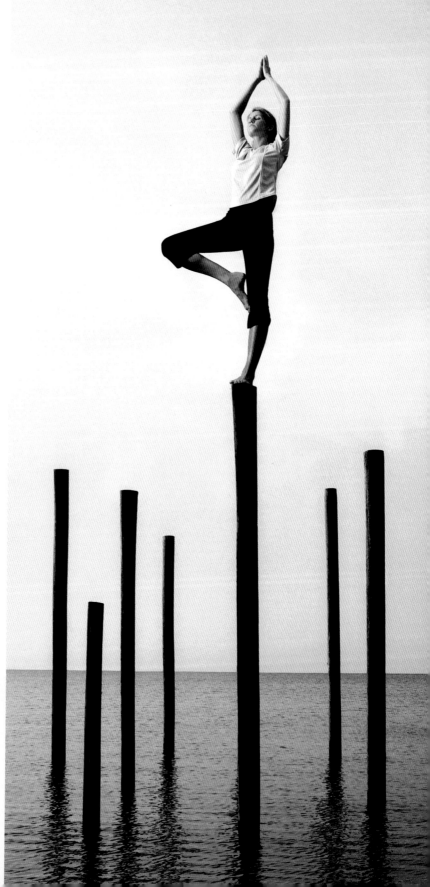

Today's yoga styles

The concepts of modern yoga are like a maze and many find them confusing to begin with. But all styles of yoga practised today can be traced back to three historical bases – religious yoga, yoga based on Patanjali's Yoga Sutras and Hatha Yoga. They all ultimately stem from the same sources, differing only in their focus. Given the variety of styles that exist, only the best-known ones will be introduced here.

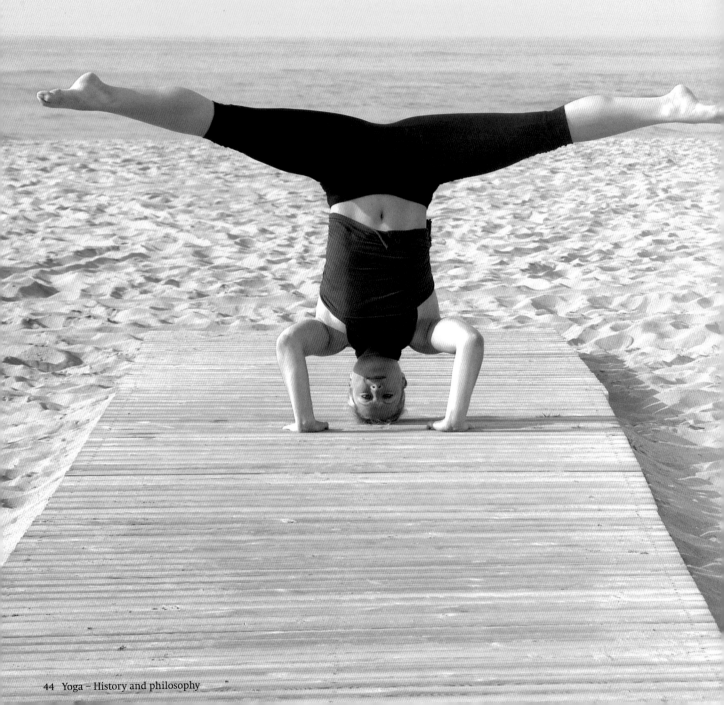

Sivananda Yoga

Sivananda Yoga started when, at the end of the 1950s, Swami Vishnudevananda (1927–93, India) was instructed by his teacher, Swami Sivananda Saraswati, to introduce yoga to the West. He opened the Sivananda Yoga Vedanta Center in Montreal, Canada, which still exists today. Sivananda centres can now be found all over the world, but predominantly in Europe and North America, where the five pillars of the Sivananda method are taught: asana practice (often referred to as the classical Hatha Yoga style) combined with breathing exercises, deep relaxation techniques, vegetarianism and meditation, combined with positive thinking.

Integral Yoga

Swami Satchidananda (1914–2002, India) was also a pupil of Swami Sivananda Saraswati. He became famous at the end of the 1960s when he encouraged thousands of spectators at the world-renowned Woodstock Music Festival to chant the holy mantra 'OM'. He opened the Integral Yoga Institute in Virginia, USA, branches of which followed worldwide. The cornerstone of his style was inherited from his teacher and involved gentle asana practice, breathing exercises, deep relaxation and meditation.

Yoga in the tradition of Tirumalai Krishnamacharya

T.K.V. Desikachar (b.late 1920s, India), son and pupil of Krishnamacharya, is the director of the Krishnamacharya Yoga Mandiram (or KYM) in Chennai (formerly Madras), India. This is a nationally renowned institution where Indian and Western pupils are still being trained today. The yoga taught in Chennai at KYM draws on the therapeutic background of Krishnamacharya, in that it concentrates on the needs of the individual, and the asana and breathing exercises are adjusted to suit the requirements and conditions of the person concerned. As a result, teaching is usually on a one-to-one basis.

Iyengar Yoga

B.K.S. Iyengar (b.1918, India), a pupil of Krishnamacharya and the uncle of Desikachar, is the founder of the Iyengar Memorial Yoga Institute in Pune (formerly Poona), India. Iyengar Yoga is one of the most famous styles of yoga and is practised worldwide. It draws on elements of the therapeutic approach, but places less emphasis on adapting the exercise sequences to the individual than on absolute precision in performing an asana. Iyengar uses numerous props to assist – blocks, belts, blankets, cushions, chairs – to enable pupils to achieve and maintain a position as accurately as possible. Only when a pupil has mastered the asana will he or she be introduced to breathing exercises. This style of yoga is energetic and highly body-oriented.

Pattabhi Jois' Ashtanga Yoga

Pattabhi Jois (b.1915, India), also a pupil of Krishnamacharya, teaches at the Ashtanga Yoga Research Institute in Karnataka (formerly Mysore), India, which was founded by him. He has mainly adopted elements of Vinyasa Yoga (see Vinyasa Yoga, p.47), which he works on refining. The distinctive feature of Ashtanga Yoga is the precise sequence of physical exercises developed by Pattabhi Jois, which has remained unchanged. In this exercise cycle – also referred to as a series – each physical posture leads on to the next. There is a progression of series, although few pupils go beyond the first series. The asanas, which are physically challenging, are practised energetically, dynamically and fluently, and are combined with breathing exercises.

Ananda Yoga

Swami Kriyananda (b.1926, Romania, of American descent) developed this style, which is also known as Kriya Yoga and is based on physical and breathing exercises developed by his teacher, Yogananda (1893–1952, USA), in 1917. They direct the energy flow to particular parts or organs of the body. This prepares the pupil for meditation and spiritual training.

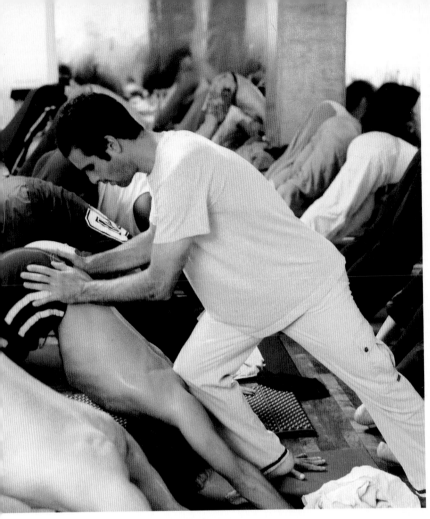

Bryan Kest, founder of Power Yoga, teaching a class.

is a synthesis of Hinduism and Islam. The Health, Happy, Holy Organization (3HO) he founded in New Mexico is now represented worldwide. Kundalini Yoga is the yoga of energy and aims to awaken kundalini, the serpent, through physical postures and breathing exercises (see p.36). Karma Yoga, the chanting of mantras, a vegetarian lifestyle and therapeutic use of yoga and Ayurveda are also part of this.

Bikram Yoga

Bikram Choudhury (b.1946, India) is happy to call himself 'Yogi to the Stars', having taught yoga to a number of Hollywood actors. He is renowned for teaching physically demanding sequences of 24 asanas combined with breathing exercises in a room heated to 30–35°C (86–95°F).

Power Yoga

Bryan Kest (b.1966, USA), a pupil of Pattabhi Jois, made the name 'Power Yoga' famous. With less focus on the spiritual, this style of yoga aims for acceptance of oneself and one's own body with highly demanding asana practice. Although pupils are meant to reach their limits during practice, they are taught to listen to their own inner teacher and not cross these, thereby achieving the greatest health benefit for body, spirit and soul.

Jivamukti Yoga

Sharon Gannon and David Life (both from the USA) developed Jivamukti Yoga, which is a spiritual style of yoga. It combines different aspects of yoga: studying the basic texts, Bhakti Yoga(see p.40), Ahimsa (see p.26), meditation and Nada Yoga (the incorporation of music, chanting and kirtan – singing of mantras – as well as the chanting of 'OM' at each lesson). Ahimsa in particular plays a central role here, which means that vegetarianism, animal welfare, environmental protection and ethical activism are included. Asana practice in the Vinyasa style is physically extremely challenging.

Kripalu Yoga

Amrit Desai is the creator of Kripula Yoga, which is based on asana practice, breathing exercises and the flowing style of Krishnamacharya. It challenges the pupil to recognize his or her own strengths and weaknesses. The asanas are practised to begin with, to ensure they are correctly performed, and movement and breathing are co-ordinated. The individual positions are then held over a prolonged period, in order to learn how to remain calmly in one position. In the third and final stage, pupils develop their own routine in which the sequence and holding of the positions depends on the needs of the pupil.

Kundalini Yoga

Yogi Bhajan (1930–2004, Pakistan) developed this style of yoga in the religious tradition of Sikhism – a religion practised in India since the end of the 15th century in which the teaching

Vinyasa Yoga

'Vinyasa Krama' more or less means 'the conscious placement of a step'. The aim is to fill the unconscious spaces between events that are consciously experienced with attentiveness and awareness.

The concept of Vinyasa Krama was adopted for the first time by Krishnamacharya in asana practice. He knew that thoughts can wander between conscious events. This can happen between individual asanas, for example, so that the next asana is anticipated, but the path leading to it is no longer experienced. To prevent this and to remain aware, centred and present at all times, Krishnamacharya co-ordinated the movement with breaths and a fluent transition from one asana to the next, so that a sort of 'meditation in motion' occurs. A logical sequence of asanas produces effects on the body, soul and spirit. This approach was continued in Ashtanga Yoga (see p.45) and is included today in numerous style movements, such as Power Yoga, Anusara Yoga and Jivamukti Yoga.

Anusara Yoga

Apart from demanding asana practice in the Vinyasa style, John Friend (b.1959, USA) above all developed a life-affirming philosophy focusing on joy and harmony that basically seeks the good in life and in all people.

The journey continues

New styles of yoga emerge almost daily, with ever-new focuses: hormone yoga, naked yoga, business yoga, acro yoga (yoga with an acrobatic bias), to name but a few. Yoga is experiencing a real boom – the whole world over! It has also grown to be of economic significance. There are yoga institutes, studios, seminars, workshops, clothes, accessories, yogi foods and much more besides. There is no end in sight to the ever-expanding world of yoga. More and more people are recognizing the wide range of benefits associated with it, because everyone can find their own style and path to inner freedom.

Workshop for one of the latest trends, acro yoga, which combines acrobatics and yoga.

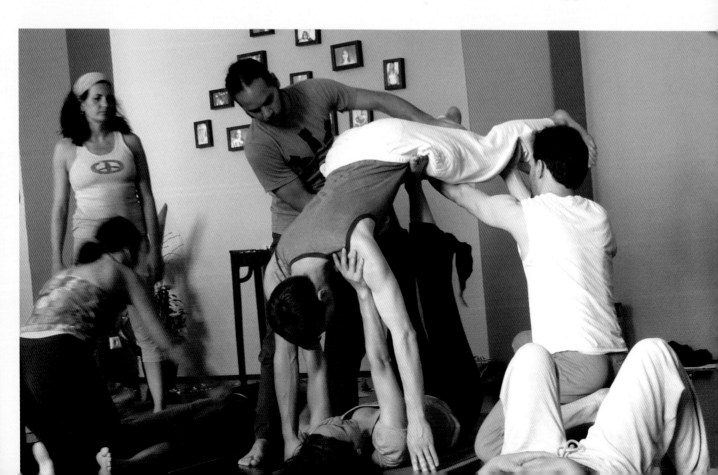

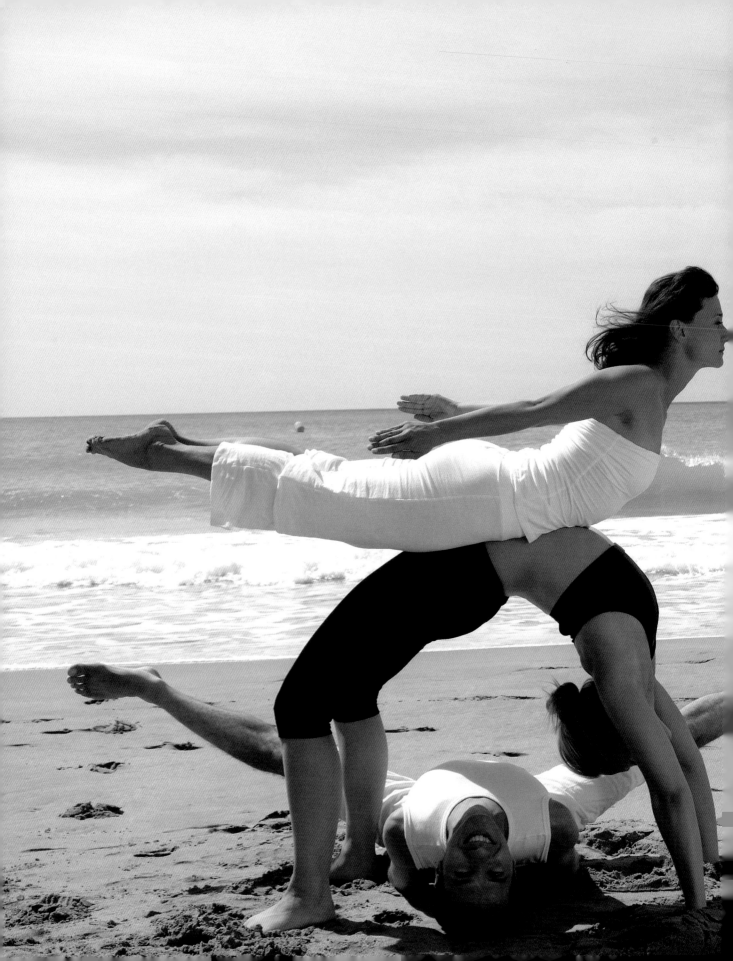

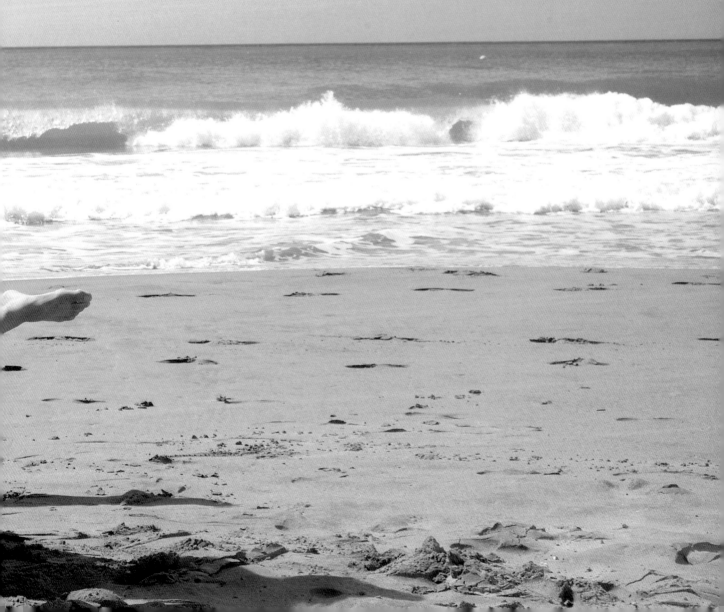

aṣanaṣ
Physical postures

EXPLANATION OF THE ASANAS

The number of different asanas

The individual postures assumed during the physical discipline of yoga are called asanas. There are reputed to be countless asanas, all of which have been developed and adapted by yogis over thousands of years.

Probably the most extensive depiction of these is contained in *The 908 Yoga Postures Master Chart* by Sri Dharma Mittra (see illustration). Sri Dharma Mittra, one of the most renowned yoga gurus in the world, compiled the poster from an original 1,350 asanas, in which he himself took the photographs. He developed 300 of the asanas, referring to himself as 'simply a body through which intuition flowed'. To date, experienced yogis have experimented with ever-new postures and the following chapters in no way claim to be comprehensive. On the contrary, the asanas selected for this book focus primarily on those taught in most yoga classes today. Although there may be variation in the way asanas are practised, depending on the style direction, the selection provides a good overview.

Asana groups

Depending on where their focal point lies, the asanas are divided into the following chapters – Sun Salutation, Standing Postures, Forward Bends, Backbends, Twists, Arm Balances, Reverse Postures, Neutral Postures and Relaxing Postures. However, some of the chapters have a mixture of asana types; for example, the chapter on standing postures also includes some backbends and forward bends.

The positive effects of asanas

The correct practice of asanas has a beneficial overall effect on physical stability, strength, flexibility and balance. It also improves blood circulation and breathing. The additional psychological effects of individual asanas will be described at the start of each section on the exercise pages.

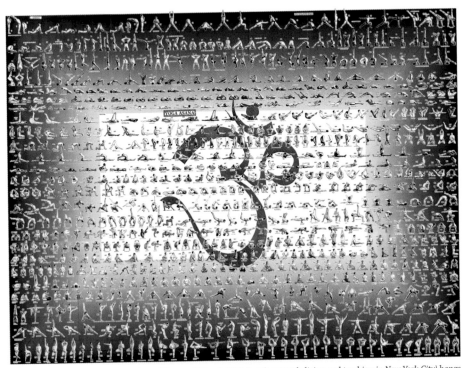

The 908 Yoga Postures Master Chart by Sri Dharma Mittra (b.1939, Brazil; currently living and teaching in New York City) hangs in many yoga studios and ashrams.

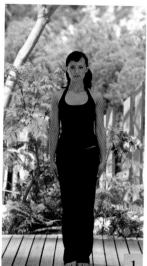
Neutral spine 1

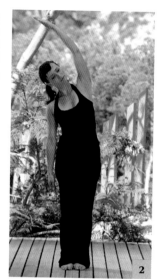
Side bend 2

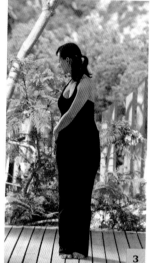
Twist 3

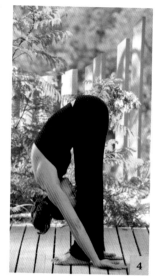
Forward bend 4

Alignment principles

The alignment of each asana is essentially based on the movement or position of the spine. This can be divided into the following five main movements:

1. Neutral spine: the spine is aligned neutrally in its natural curve.
2. Side bend: the spine is stretched to the side.
3. Twist: the spine is turned around its own axis.
4. Forward bend: the spine bends forward from the pelvis; the back of the body is stretched.
5. Backbend: the spine bends back from the chest; the front of the body is stretched.

Stability and effortlessness

The yogi tries to find stability and effortlessness in equal measure in each asana, in other words, he tries to remain stably aligned and firmly rooted during the asana and at the same time achieve a feeling of ease. This feeling enables him to maintain the posture without exerting himself beyond his own limits, and to hold it for a short time to begin with, then for longer as he practises more. The crucial element assisting him in this is breathing. As long as he can breathe calmly and evenly during an asana, a feeling of effortlessness will prevail. As a result, breathing is also referred to as the inner teacher who must be listened to over and over again. Other aids that make practising asanas easier are shown on p.52.

Nobody is perfect

Each asana is by its nature 'empty' – equally difficult or easy. What one person finds difficult, another may find easy. Everyone has their own strengths and weaknesses, preferences and inclinations. Do not become disheartened, but instead try to approach each asana with a new and fresh perspective. And do not be put off by the apparent complexity and degree of difficulty of an asana. Nobody is perfect and everyone has to start somewhere. Just keep practising.

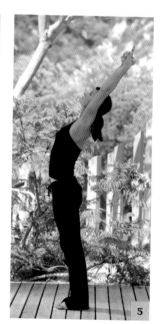
Backbend 5

Movement and counter-movement

A further principle of each asana involves the extension of the body through movement and counter-movement. Different body parts are affected by this, depending on the asana. If you press your heels down firmly while standing, the top of your head will be drawn up; if you push your heels forward while sitting, your tailbone moves back. But the point is always to turn your body in different directions, in order to create space even in the most complex positions.

Asana aids

Bandhas: The body's locks

Bandha (from the Sanskrit for 'lock' or 'seal') refers to the body's locks, which control and direct energy within the body like a valve. Setting the bandhas and using them effectively in the asana as a support or even as a prop requires some practice. Firstly, the bandhas are subtle muscle contractions and, secondly, greater concentration is needed to set and hold them.

Mula bandha

Mula bandha (*Mula* meaning 'root' or 'base' in Sanskrit) gives strength and stability. In addition, it prevents the pelvis from tipping back and producing a hollow back. In order to perform Mula bandha, the pelvic floor is contracted while inhaling. This causes the tailbone to move down and forward, so the sacral bone is pulled down and the lower back is elongated. This stabilizes the lumbar vertebrae and prevents bad posture in the lower back. The muscle contraction lies primarily in the perineum (the space between the anus and the genitals). To begin with, it helps to imagine wanting to go to the toilet but being unable to, as this activates the anal sphincter. The ability to isolate and contract the perineal muscles develops in time.

Uddiyana bandha

Uddiyana bandha (*uddiyana* from the Sanskrit for 'to fly upwards') stabilizes the central and upper back. This prevents bad posture, particularly around the thoracic

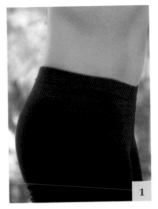
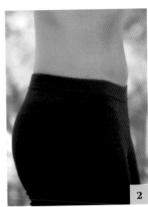

Mula bandha: relaxed   *Mula bandha: tensed*

vertebrae. To perform Uddiyana bandha, the lower abdomen is pulled in during exhalation and the navel is drawn upwards. This creates a slight vacuum in the ribcage and an upward pull; both produce a certain feeling of lightness.

Holding Mula bandha and Uddiyana bandha

To achieve a combined effect of stability and effortlessness, Mula bandha is performed on the inhalation and Uddiyana bandha on the exhalation. To begin with it is not easy to maintain the concentration needed in order to perform bandhas, but with a little practice they become almost second nature.

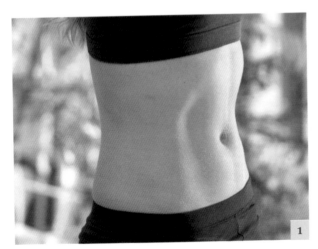

Uddiyana bandha: relaxed

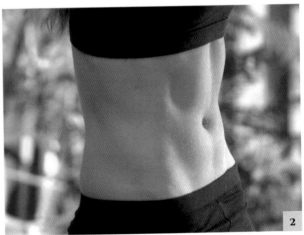

Uddiyana bandha: tensed

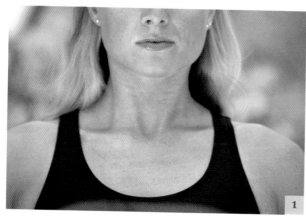

Jalandhara bandha: relaxed

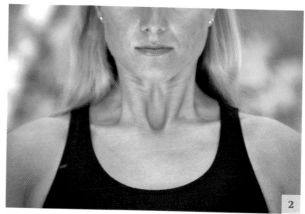

Jalandhara bandha: tensed

Jalandhara bandha

Jalandhara bandha (*jalandhara* from the Sanskrit for 'net' or 'tissue') controls the energy flow between the heart and the brain and prevents pressure on the heart. It is mainly performed during breathing exercises, particularly while the breath is controlled (see pranayama chapter, pp.216–23), when the neck vertebrae are extended up, the chin is lowered slightly and the larynx drawn in gently.

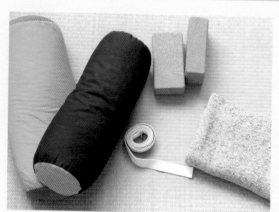

Props: Cushions, wooden blocks, belt and blanket

Other props

If you are unable to reach the floor or it is too hard, good stability will not be achieved or there will be insufficient mobility for correct alignment. This is when the use of props, such as a belt, cushion, block (wooden or foam) or blanket, is useful. These help you to become correctly aligned in individual positions and to develop a feel for what the asana involves. Each asana includes a description of how the props should be used.

Namaste and drishti: Improvers of concentration

Namaste in Sanskrit roughly means: 'The divinity in me bows to the divinity in you'. This gesture is often used as a greeting, when taking one's leave and as a thank-you. It also improves concentration on an asana.

Drishti means 'gaze' in Sanskrit and denotes a point of focus where the gaze rests. It does not mean focusing on an actual object, but rather supporting movement with the direction of the gaze and protecting the consciousness from distractions. The inner as well as the outer gaze follows the movement.

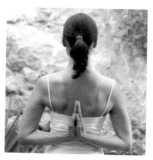

Namaste at the back

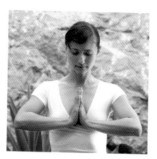

Namaste on the chest

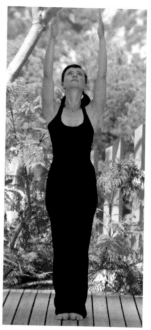

Drishti: Direction of the gaze

How an asana page is set out

Notes on the different elements

Name of the asana
in Sanskrit

Each asana is
illustrated and
described in
detail. Particular
attention is paid
to alignment in
a posture, so that
it is properly
understood and
practised correctly
right from the
start. The way in
which breathing
can assist with
the asana is also
indicated.

utthita parsvakonasana Extended Side Angle Pose

This asana strengthens the ankles, knees and thighs. At the same time, the side of the body is stretched along its entire length and the hips are opened. This posture improves digestion and alleviates sciatica and arthritis.

Alignment

- Lunge back and turn your back foot to an angle of 90 degrees. Your front foot should be pointing forward.
- Stretch your back leg, taking the weight on the outer edge of the foot and turn the thigh out slightly.
- Bend your front leg, so that the shin is vertical and the thigh is parallel to the ground.
- Place the hand of your lower arm flat on the ground, on the outer edge of the front foot, and support your weight with the whole of your hand. Your knee should press out towards this arm.
- Stretch your upper arm over your head, lengthening your body diagonally and forward. Your whole body should produce a line from the foot of your straight leg to the fingertips of your hand on the same side. Your weight should be evenly distributed on both legs and the front hand.
- Inhale and stretch from your fingertips to the toes of your back foot.
- Look up and lower your pelvis further into the posture.

For beginners

Rest your lower arm on your thigh and stretch your upper arm over your head, so that your body forms a line.

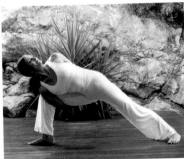

For beginners

If you cannot reach the floor, place a block under your hand.

baddha parsvakonasana
Bound Extended Side Angle Pose

This asana has the same effect as Utthita Parsvakonasana. It also includes a shoulder stretch, which opens the shoulders further. This has a positive effect on breathing and improves breathing volume.

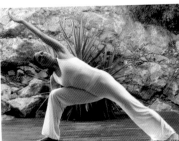

Rear view detail

For beginners

Place your hand flat on the ground to the inside of your front foot, taking your weight through your whole foot. Stretch your upper arm behind your back and place your hand on your bent thigh. ▼

Alignment

- Assume Utthita Parsvakonasana (see p.86).
- From this position, extend your lower arm beneath your bent thigh and take the upper arm behind your back. Grab your fingers or, if possible, the wrist of your upper arm (see rear view detail).
- Exhale and rotate your body to the side, pushing your tailbone back.
- Look up towards the sky.

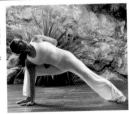

Translation of the
asana

The way in which
the asana works
and its effects
on the body are
described in
detail.

Photos showing
detailed close-ups
or those taken
from different
perspectives help
provide a deeper
understanding of
each asana.

With many asanas, simpler alternatives are shown for beginners, either with or without props, so that even novices can benefit from the positive effects of the postures.

ardha chandrasana Half Moon Pose

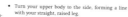

Half Moon Pose strengthens the abdomen, back, buttocks, thighs and ankles. It also strengthens the lumbar vertebrae and the sacrum, and alleviates sciatica. It promotes a sense of balance, creating a feeling of steadiness and stability.

Alignment

- Find a firm position on your supporting leg and distribute your weight over your entire foot. Your foot should be pointing straight in front.
- Place your hand like a tent roughly 30cm (12 inches) in front of your supporting foot, lift your other leg up and extend it straight back.
- Straighten your supporting leg and press it firmly into the floor. Straighten your raised leg and push it backwards, making sure your toes are flexed. The foot of your raised leg should be parallel with the floor.
- Open out your hips and turn both thighs out slightly.

- Turn your upper body to the side, forming a line with your straight, raised leg.
- Keep your shoulders relaxed and open as your arms form a vertical line.
- Inhale and stretch forward through the crown of your head and back through your raised foot. Your tailbone should be stretched towards your raised ankle.
- Exhale and twist further to the side, stretching your upper arm gently upwards and your lower arm down. The lower arm should act as a stabilizer but should barely carry any weight.
- Look up towards your extended arm. If you cannot hold your balance, look down.

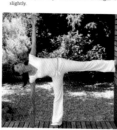

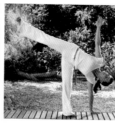

For beginners
Place your lower hand on a block and press the foot of your raised leg firmly against a wall.

For advanced students
Place your front hand flat on the floor. This will cause your upper body to tilt down further. Extend your raised leg higher, so that your leg and upper body are in line again.

With many asanas, alternatives for advanced students are also shown, so that even the more experienced can constantly find new challenges and thereby improve their practice.

dwi pada rajakapotasana Double Pigeon Pose

This asana has the same effect as Baddha Konasana (opposite). It opens and stretches the hips and knees, but even more intensely. With a little practice, this asana can be used to solve stubborn tensions in the buttocks.

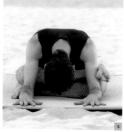

Step-by-Step alignment

1. Get into a seated position. Bend one leg and position it so that your shin bone is parallel to the floor in front of you. Bend your other leg and rest the knee on the ankle of your lower foot and place the upper ankle on the knee of your lower leg.
2. As you inhale, stretch your arms upwards and pull your spine up through the crown of your head.
3. Exhale and bend from the hips as far forward as you can, pushing your tailbone back at the same time. Your back should remain straight. Place your arms in front of you and relax your neck.

- Keep your breathing even and try to relax your hips as far as possible.

▼ For beginners

a. If you find that you cannot open your hips very far, lay your shin bones one in front of the other.

b. Alternatively, stretch one leg out, bend your other leg and lay the outer ankle bone on the lower knee.

c. If you cannot lower your knee to your inside ankle bone, place a cushion between your knee and your ankle bone.

Make sure your shins are straight in front of you and lie parallel on top of each other.

Where necessary, particularly in the case of more complex asanas, step-by-step descriptions with accompanying photographs show how the posture is achieved and what the correct alignment should be.

The exclamation mark is used to highlight special aspects of the asana, which must be noted. This may be a tip to practise or a warning that special care is needed. Or it may be that the previous postures should first be mastered before the asana is attempted.

Preparatory exercises

Before you start your asana practice, it is important to mobilize your body, particularly the joints and spine. There are numerous exercises that loosen up the body. Combine the following preparatory exercises to suit yourself and your own needs.

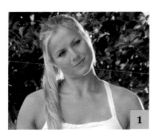

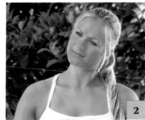

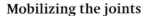

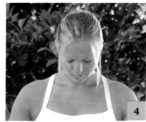

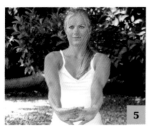

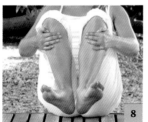

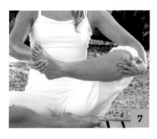

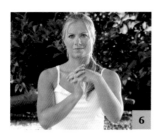

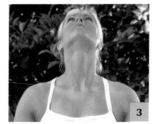

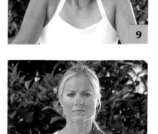

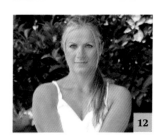

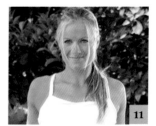

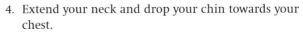

Mobilizing the joints

Sit in a comfortable position, possibly on a cushion, so that you can align your spine.

1. Tilt your head gently to the right.
2. Next tilt your head gently to the left.
3. Allow your head to fall back without bending your neck vertebrae.
4. Extend your neck and drop your chin towards your chest.
5. Interlace your fingers and stretch your arms out in front of you; your elbows will turn in slightly.
6. Bend your elbows and interlace your fingers, gently rotating your wrist joints in both directions.
7. Begin by taking hold of one of your bent legs under the knee and by the foot and gently rotating the foot; move both hands to your knee and turn the knee joint. Repeat with your other leg.
8. Draw circles in the air with your raised feet, changing direction.
9. Raise your shoulders as far as you can.
10. Lower your shoulders completely.
11. Pull your shoulders back, without causing your back to hollow.
12. Pull your shoulders forward, without rounding your back.

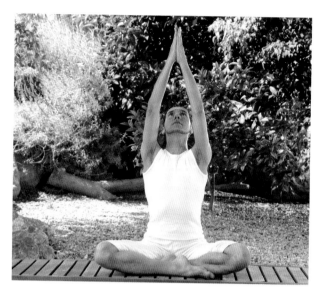

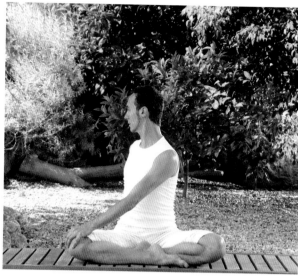

Sit comfortably upright with your legs crossed, so that you can straighten your spine. If this is uncomfortable, sit on a cushion. Inhale and raise your arms up.

As you exhale, turn to the right. Place your right hand close to your tailbone and lay your left hand lightly on your right thigh. Don't force the turn with your hands. Change sides and repeat the exercise.

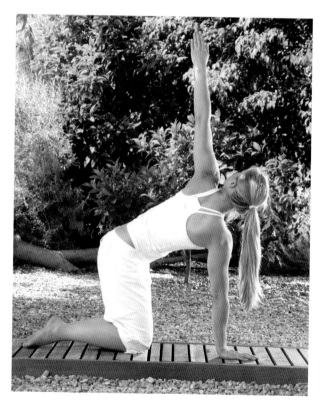

Mobilizing the spine: Twisting

The mobilization exercises on this page are intended to prepare the spine for a twist. The body twists on its own axis and the spine remains straight here too. The hips remain parallel.

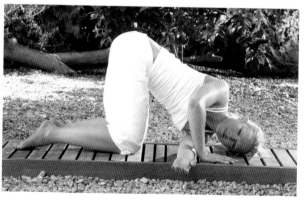

Go onto all fours, i.e. onto your hands and knees. Align your hips above your knees and your shoulders above your wrists. Inhale and gently raise one arm out to the side and up.

As you exhale, bring your outstretched arm under the other side of your body and lower your shoulder onto the floor, placing your arm behind your supporting hand. Repeat this exercise a few times on both sides.

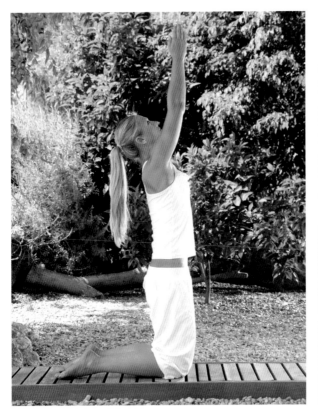

Preparatory exercises

Mobilizing the spine: Stretching and bending

These mobilization exercises prepare the spine for forward bends and backbends. The spine is stretched and bent along its entire length, while the hips remain parallel.

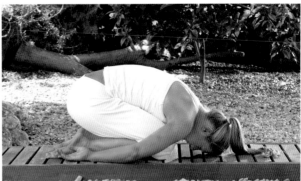

While in the kneeling position, inhale and raise your hands upwards. Your hips should be aligned above your knees. Stretch up from your thoracic vertebrae and gently tilt your pelvis forward, to avoid hollowing your back.

As you exhale, bend your upper body forward over your thighs, sit on your heels, turn your forehead to the floor and place your arms (palms facing up) back alongside your body. Lengthen the nape of your neck through your rounded back and tuck your tailbone under. Repeat the exercise a few times.

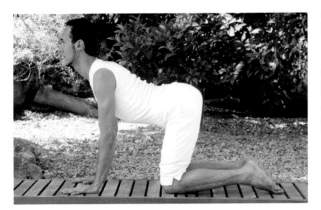

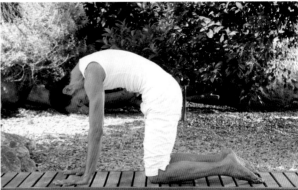

Go onto all fours, i.e. onto your hands and knees, and align your shoulders above your wrists and your hips above your knees. The soles of your feet should face upwards. While inhaling, lengthen your spine and direct your gaze slightly upwards.

As you exhale, round your back into Cat Pose and pull your tailbone in. Direct your gaze in towards your body, so that your entire spine is rounded. Repeat the exercise a few times.

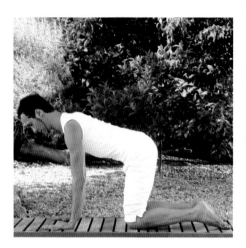

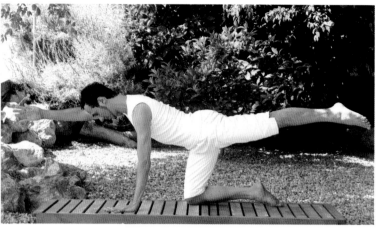

Go onto all fours, keeping your spine straight. Align your shoulders directly above your wrists and your hips above your knees.

Inhale and bring one arm forward and the opposite leg back. Hold this position for several breaths. On inhaling, extend your outstretched arm forward and your leg back, so that your body is gently stretched diagonally. Your neck should remain a natural extension of your spine and your gaze should be directed downwards. Repeat on the opposite side.

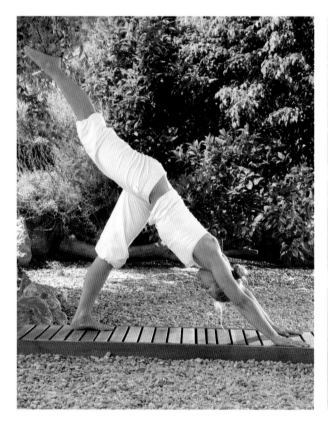

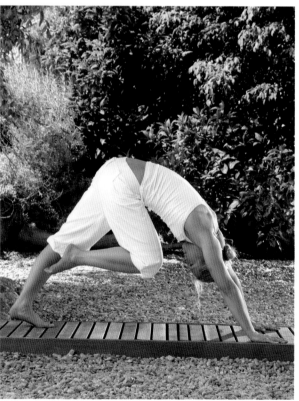

From Adho Mukha Svanasana (see p.67), raise one leg up while inhaling, and stretch along the body from your fingertips to your toes. Press from your shoulders through your arms and keep your hips parallel.

Exhale and draw your knee in towards your nose, at the same time arching your spine. Your neck should be a continuation of your curved spine and your gaze should be directed towards your knee.

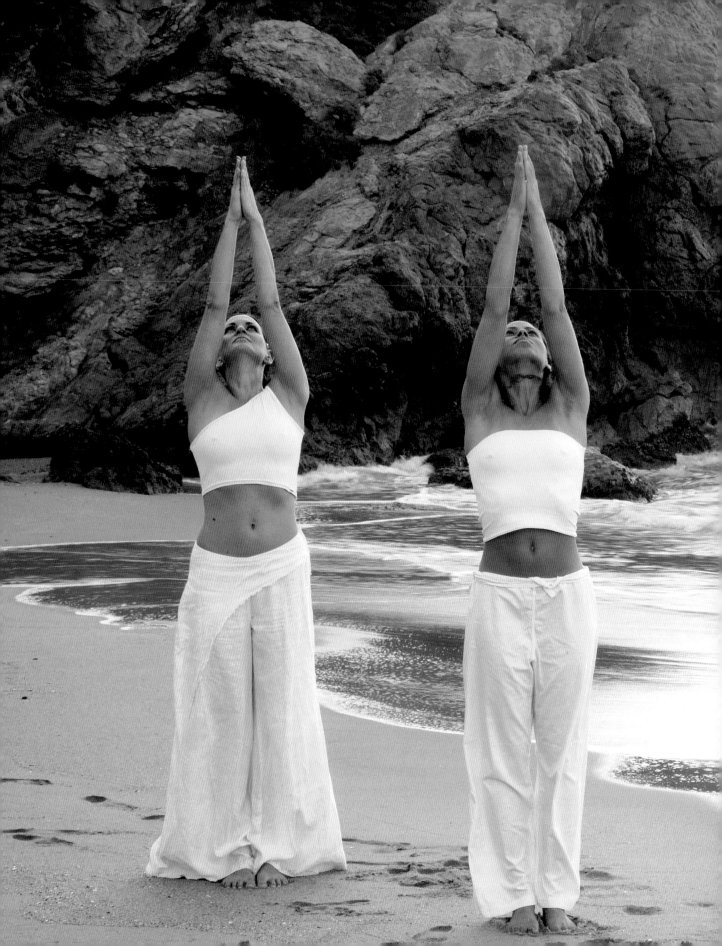

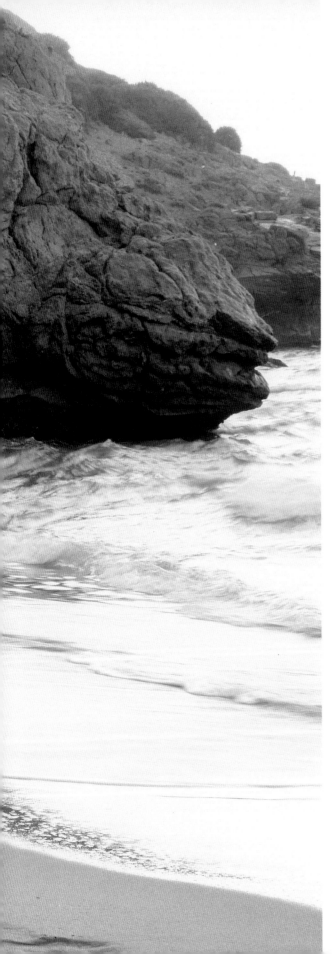

Sun Salutation

The Sun Salutation (Surya Namaskar) involves a sequence of exercises that were traditionally performed in India before or at sunrise. Of course it can be practised at any time of the day and is an ideal warm-up at the start of a yoga session. The spine and all the joints, muscles, tendons and ligaments are stretched and elongated, so that the entire body is mobilized. The exercises are performed in rapid succession and co-ordinated with the breath. Many repeat the Sun Salutation a number of times at an increasing speed, until the body is completely warmed up and perfectly prepared for more asana practice.

There are numerous variations of the Sun Salutation, but they are all based on two classical sequences – Surya Namaskar A and B. These are introduced and explained on the following pages.

surya namaskar a   Sun Salutation A

Sun Salutation A is a classical yoga sequence and includes exercises that can easily be learned by heart. It is an excellent way of warming up before a yoga session and can also be used as a short exercise in between, as the whole body is mobilized, stretched, elongated and strengthened. Each individual asana making up the Sun Salutation is described in detail and explained on the following pages.

Sun Salutation

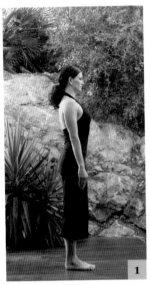

Starting posture: Tadasana, see p.64

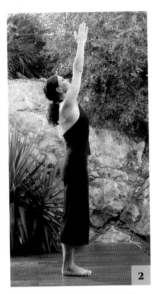

IN in Urdhva Hastasana, see p.64

Points to remember

- Co-ordinate the individual asanas with your breathing and move smoothly and dynamically from one posture to the next.

- The photo captions indicate when you should inhale and exhale (IN = inhale, EX = exhale).

- Try to inhale or exhale a fraction of a second before the movement.

- Your inhalation and exhalation should be of equal length.

- Adjust your movement according to the length of your breath, so that movement and breathing come together as one.

- Practise the Sun Salutation slowly to begin with, so that you warm up properly.

The Sun Salutation can be genuinely challenging at first, but with a little practice your breaths will become calmer, more even and longer – and your movements will be more flexible.

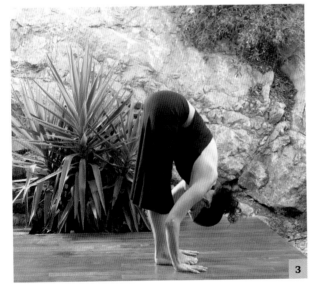

EX in Uttanasana, see p.65

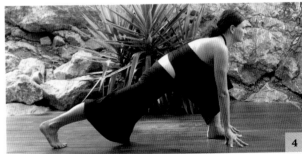

IN during the lunge, see p.66

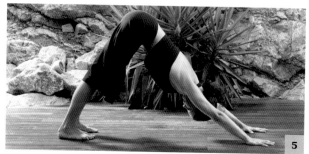

EX in Adho Mukha Svanasana, see p.67 **5**

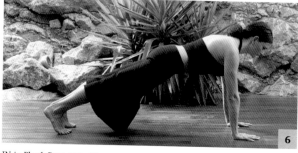

IN in Plank Pose, see p.68 **6**

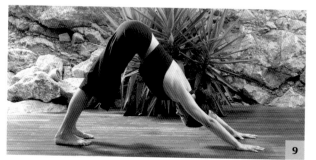

EX in Knees, Chest and Chin, see p.69 **7**

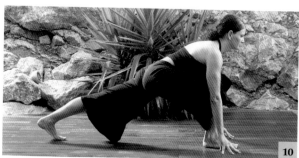

IN in Bhujangasana, see p.70 **8**

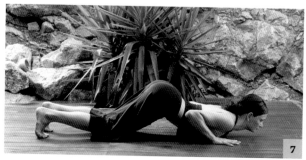

EX in Adho Mukha Svanasana, see p.67 **9**

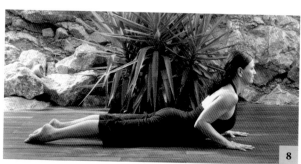

IN during the lunge, see p.66 **10**

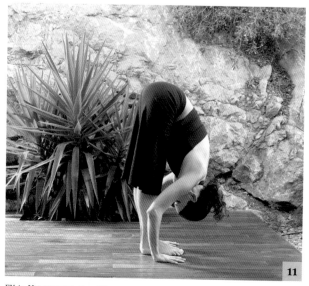

EX in Uttanasana, see p.65 **11**

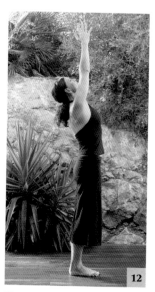

12

IN in Urdhva Hastasana, see p.64

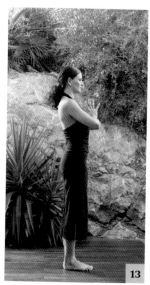

13

EX in Tadasana, see p.64

tadasana Mountain Pose
urdhva hastasana Extended Mountain Pose

Mountain Pose is a characteristically straight, upright and steady pose. The spine is stretched and the muscles straightening the trunk are strengthened, as are the leg, abdominal and shoulder muscles. This improves overall body posture and creates an awareness of when the spine is correctly aligned.

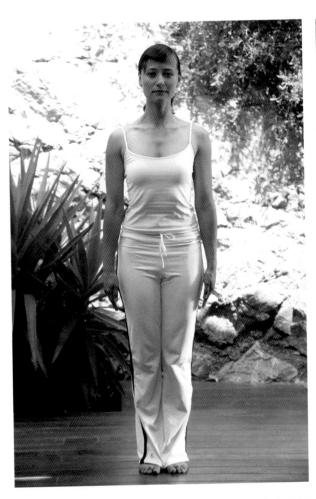

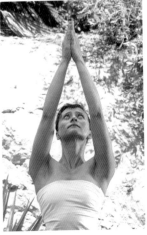

◀ **Urdhva Hastasana**

Inhale and raise your hands together from Tadasana above your head. Your gaze should follow your hands. Hold the body's alignment in Tadasana; apart from the arms, the head should be slightly raised and the upper back should not arch back.

Alignment

- Stand up straight and bring your feet together. Spread your weight evenly across your feet. Make sure your toes are flat to the floor and slightly splayed.

- Draw your kneecaps up slightly and gently tense the thigh muscles.

- Move your pelvis to the neutral position. Tuck your tailbone under and raise your pubic bone.

- Draw your navel in towards your spine, so that the abdominal muscles are slightly tensed.

- Stretch your spine upwards and allow your shoulders and upper arms to drop away. Turn your forearms in.

- Lengthen your neck by raising the crown of your head upwards and bringing your chin in towards your chest slightly.

- Look straight ahead.

Finding Tadasana

The alignment principle of Tadasana is the basis of almost every posture: strength and stability in the legs, a straight, elongated spine and a feeling of effortlessness, through the lengthening of the spine up through the crown of the head.

uttanasana Standing Forward Bend
urdhva uttanasana Deep Forward Fold

This asana gives the spine and hamstrings a really good, gentle stretch while the lower back is relaxed. The pose has a calming effect overall and helps with negative moods. It also controls blood pressure, improves blood supply to the brain and alleviates stomach and back pain.

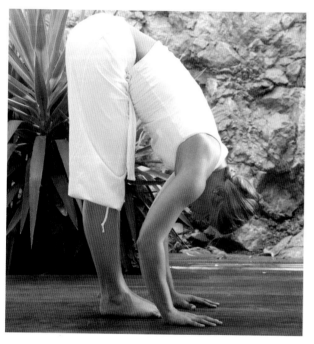

Alignment

- Bend your upper body forward from the hips and draw your hamstrings and tailbone upwards.

- Drop your shoulder blades away from your ears towards your hips.

- Spread your hands flat on the floor, bending your legs if necessary, and lengthen your neck and lower back.

- Inhale and lower the crown of your head; exhale and draw your upper body towards your legs.

- Look towards your legs.

- Exhale as you go into the asana and inhale as you come out of it.

▼ **Urdhva Uttanasana**

On inhaling come out of Uttanasana onto your fingertips or a block and stretch your back forward. This position is also good as a beginner's version of Uttanasana.

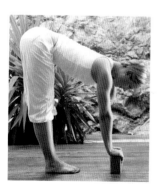

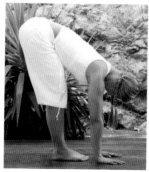

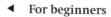

For advanced students ▶

Place your hands flat on the ground either side of your feet. On the exhalation, lower your upper body to your thighs and draw your nose in towards your knees.

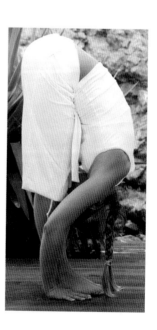

◀ **For beginners**

If you cannot lay your hands flat, bend your knees slightly.

Asanas – Physical postures 65

Lunge

In the lunge, the spine, the front thigh muscle on the straight leg and the hamstring on the bent leg are all lengthened and stretched. The hip flexor muscles are stretched alternately and the shoulders are opened up. This asana, which has no Sanskrit name, is used primarily as a warm-up and as a transition between postures.

Alignment

- Bend your front leg to a maximum of 90 degrees, position your knee above your ankle and press the back of your leg down into your heel.
- Place the palms of both hands down firmly on either side of your front foot.
- Let your tailbone drop down, keeping your hips parallel.
- Open up your shoulders, turn your upper arms in slightly and extend your neck to lengthen your spine.
- Inhale as you assume the posture and exhale as you come out of it.

Transitions:

From Uttanasana (see p.65)

Inhale and stretch one leg right back, while bending your front leg. Place your hands down on either side of your front foot.

From Adho Mukha Svanasana (see p.67)

Inhale and bring your back foot in between your hands. Reach back with one hand if you cannot get the foot between your hands.

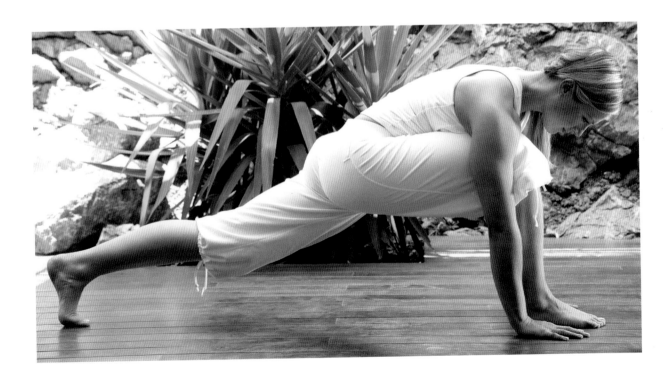

अधो मुख श्वानासन adho mukha svanasana Downward Facing Dog Pose

In Downward Facing Dog Pose the whole back is stretched, and the shoulders are opened and become looser. The legs, ankles, arms and wrists are similarly strengthened. The pose stimulates the nervous system and supplies the body with fresh energy.

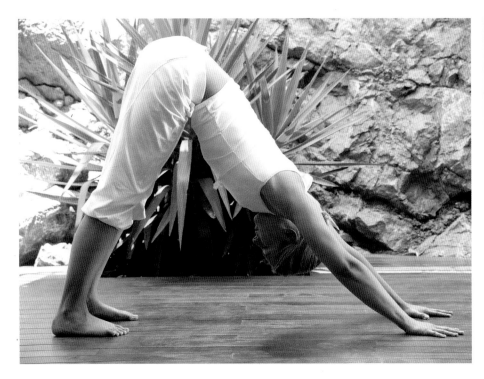

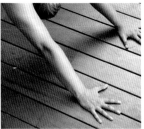

Detailed view ▲

Spread your fingers out and make sure that your whole hand is taking your weight by pressing your finger joints into the floor. Your middle finger should point straight ahead.

Alignment

- Place your feet hip-width apart.
- Your feet should be parallel to each other. Press your ankles down into the floor.
- Stretch your legs and press your thighs back.
- Push your buttocks, tailbone and sit bones upwards.
- Lengthen your back from the lumbar vertebrae to the neck.
- Open up your shoulders and turn your upper arms out and your underarms in (see detailed view of hands).
- Relax your neck and look towards your navel.
- Distribute your weight evenly between your hands and feet.
- Assume the asana while exhaling and come out of it while inhaling.

If your heels cannot touch the floor, place a blanket under them.

chatturanga dandasana   Yogic Push-up Pose

This asana strengthens the whole body – from the wrists, through the arms, abdomen and back muscles to the legs. At the same time the ribcage is expanded. It works against lethargy and tiredness and instils a feeling of strength and freshness.

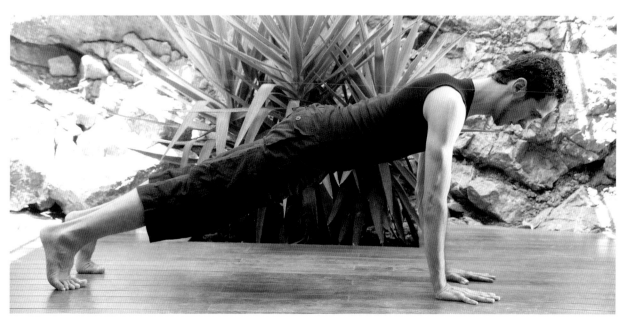

Starting posture: Plank Pose

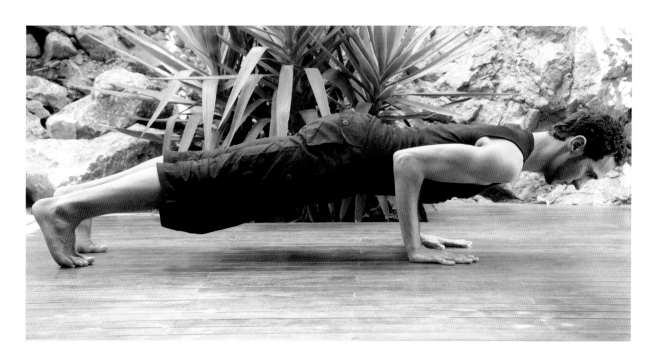

Alignment

- While inhaling, assume the Plank Pose (see Starting posture).
- Tense your leg muscles and push your heels down.
- Spread your fingers out, taking the weight through the whole hand, and stretch your arms. Your shoulders should be positioned above your wrists. Turn your upper arms out slightly.
- Inhale and lengthen your spine. Your neck should remain straight, lengthening the spine, and your body should form a straight line.
- On the exhalation, lower your body powerfully. Tense your entire body, particularly your abdominal muscles, so that your back does not sag.
- Your upper and lower arms should be at 90 degrees to each other. Press your upper arms in towards your ribs.
- Pull your shoulder blades back. Your shoulders and elbows should form a line.
- Direct your gaze at the floor.

For beginners

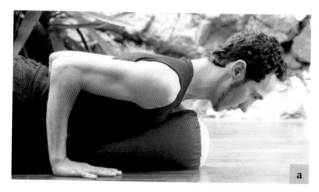

a. Chatturanga Dandasana with cushion

If your arms are not yet strong enough, lay a cushion under your body lengthways to support your weight. This is a particularly good way of practising the correct body and, in particular, arm position.

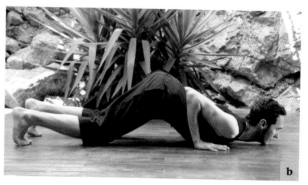

b. Knees, Chest and Chin

The Knees, Chest and Chin variant can be practised to build up strength in the arms and also to warm up:

- First lower your knees, then your chest and finally your chin to the floor.
- Push your pelvis up and press your hands firmly onto the ground with your fingers spread out. Look forward.

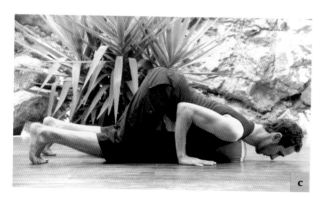

c. Knees, Chest and Chin with cushion

This variant is suitable for developing a feel for the correct alignment, even if you are not yet strong enough to hold the posture.

Chatturanga Dandasana requires a great deal of energy and body tension. If your lower back is not strong enough, this can lead to back problems, so practise the alternatives first.

bhujaṅgāsana Cobra Pose

This asana, also known as Serpent Pose, opens the chest and stretches the shoulders. The back muscles, legs and spine are strengthened, particularly the thoracic vertebrae. This pose has an invigorating effect on the mind and body and relieves tension in the upper back.

Alignment

- Lie on your front with the tops of your feet flat and press them down into the floor.
- Relax your buttocks and press your outstretched legs, hips and pubic bone into the floor.
- Inhale and lengthen your spine, gently lifting your breastbone.
- Place your hands beneath your shoulders and gently 'push' the floor forwards.
- Tuck your elbows into your body and gently pull them back.

- Look straight ahead without allowing your head to sink into your neck.
- Assume the pose on the inhalation and release it on the exhalation.

For beginners

a. If your back is still a little stiff, bend your arms more.

b. Or place your hands further in front of you and pull up from here through your breastbone.

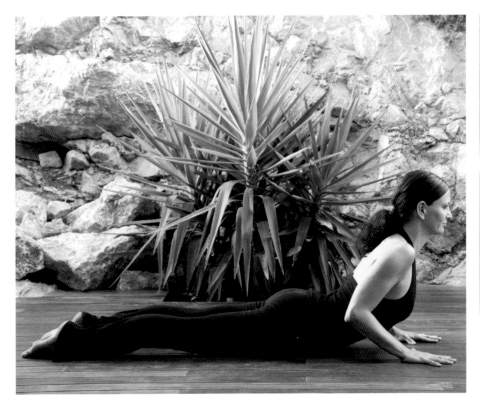
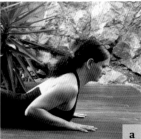
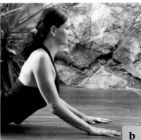

उर्ध्व मुख स्वनासन Upward Facing Dog Pose

In this posture the chest is fully opened and the shoulders are stretched. The stomach and leg muscles are also strengthened and the whole back becomes more flexible. Opening the chest not only has a beneficial effect on the lungs, but also lifts the spirits.

Alignment

- Lie on your front with your soles facing upwards and press the tops of your feet firmly into the ground.

- Tense your leg and stomach muscles and draw your tailbone under slightly. Raise your legs off the ground, so that only the tops of your feet are touching the ground.

- As you inhale, bend your entire upper body back with your chest open, extending the backbend right through the spine.

- Tilt your pelvis forward slightly to avoid a hollow back.

- Position your wrists directly below your shoulders and push yourself up. Make sure your whole hand takes the weight. Your wrist and arm should form a right angle.

- Turn your shoulders out slightly and turn your underarms in.

- Look up making sure that your neck remains an extension of your spine.

- Inhale as you go into the posture; exhale as you come out.

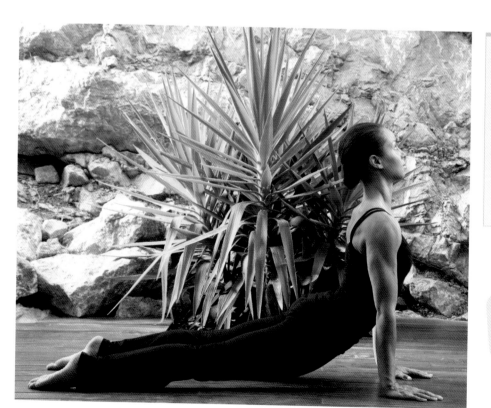

Transition from Chatturanga Dandasana (see p.68)

Push yourself back slightly on your hands and turn your feet so that they are pointing back. Inhale and move forward and up, keeping your legs off the ground.

Upward Facing Dog is a very intense pose. Begin by practising the Cobra (see p.70).

surya namaskar b Sun Salutation B

Surya Namaskar B is a challenging variant of the Sun Salutation. It can be practised following Sun Salutation A (see Points to remember, p.62). The more advanced student will be able to go straight into Sun Salutation B as their warm-up.

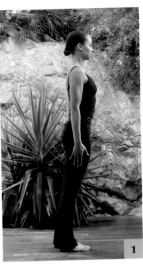

1

Starting posture: Tadasana, see p.64

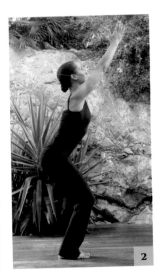

2

IN in Utkatasana, see p.81

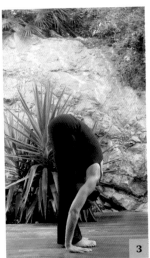

3

EX in Uttanasana, see p.65

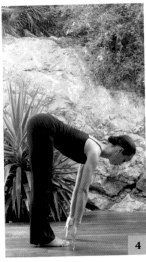

4

IN in Urdhva Uttanasana, see p.65

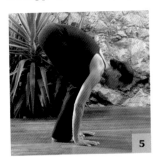

5

Hold your breath and jump into Chatturanga, see p.74

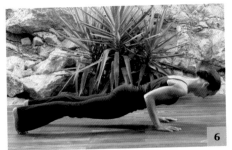

6

EX in Chatturanga, see p.68

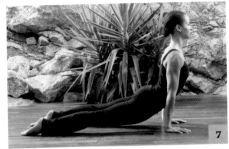

7

IN in Urdhva Mukha Svanasana, see p.71

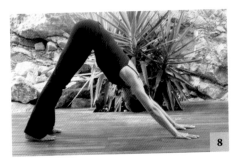

8

EX in Adho Mukha Svanasana, see p.67

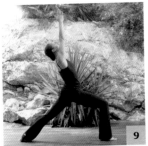

9

IN in Virabhadrasana I (right leg forward), see p.78

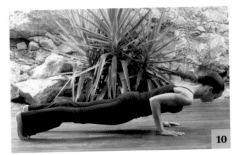

10

EX in Chatturanga, see p.68

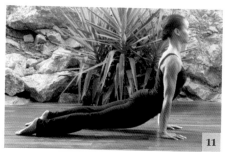

IN in Urdhva Mukha Svanasana, see p.71

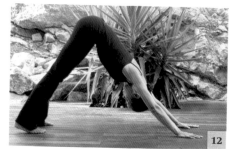

EX in Adho Mukha Svanasana, see p.67

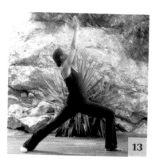

IN in Virabhadrasana I
(left leg forward), see p.78

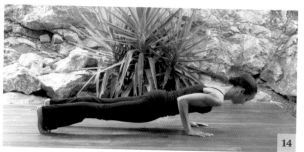

EX in Chatturanga, see p.68

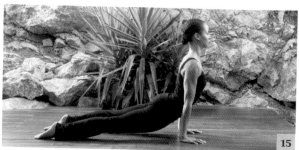

IN in Urdhva Mukha Svanasana, see p.71

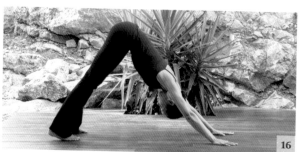

EX in Adho Mukha Svanasana, see p.67

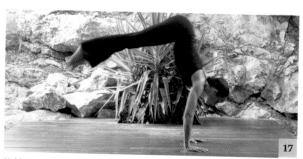

Hold your breath and jump into Urdhva Uttanasana, see p.75

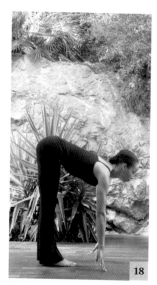

IN in Urdhva Uttanasana,
see p.65

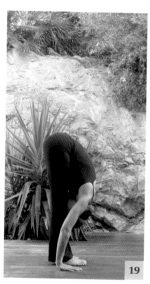

EX in Uttanasana, see p.65

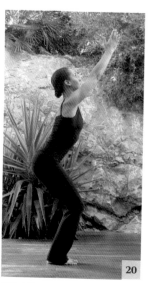

IN in Utkatasana, see p.81

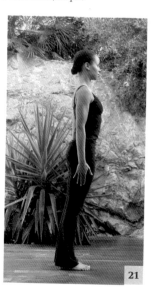

EX in Tadasana, see p.64

Jump from Urdhva Uttanasana into Chatturanga Dandasana

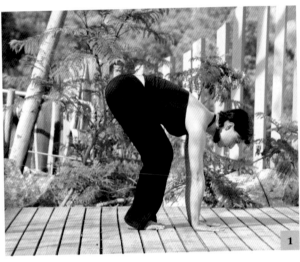

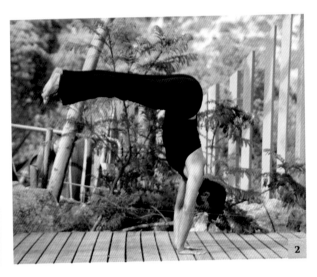

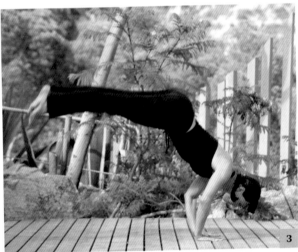

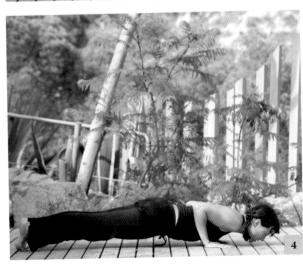

Step-by-step jumping into the postures

1. Inhale in Urdhva Uttanasana (see p.65) and hold your breath briefly while bending your legs. Place your hands flat on the ground and spread out your fingers. Distribute your weight evenly through your hands.

2. Perform Mula bandha (see p.52) and tense your abdominal muscles. Push off from your legs and push your buttocks up as far as possible, so that your body forms a right angle.

3. From here push your legs back, maintaining the tension throughout your entire body.

4. Land with bent Chatturanga Dandasana arms, cushioning your landing with your entire body, not just your back. Keep your leg and abdominal muscles firm to prevent your back from sagging and your spine from having to take the weight. Exhale in Chatturanga Dandasana (see p.68).

Jumping from Adho Mukha Svanasana into Urdhva Uttanasana

Step-by-step jumping into the postures

1. Exhale in Adho Mukha Svanasana (see p.67), hold your breath briefly and bend your legs. Look forward.

2. Perform Uddiyana bandha (see p.52). Shift your weight onto your hands and push up and forward from your legs. Draw your buttocks up as far as possible, so that your body forms a right angle.

3. Now draw your stretched legs into your body with your arms remaining straight.

4. Land with your feet as close as possible to your hands and breathe in Urdhva Uttansana (see p.65).

Jumps require precise alignment and a certain amount of body control, and should only be attempted when you have some practical experience. Apart from the correct technique, you also need quite strong arm, leg and abdominal muscles. If jumps are practised incorrectly, they can lead to back problems, particularly close to the lumbar vertebrae. Jumps should be approached slowly and patiently.

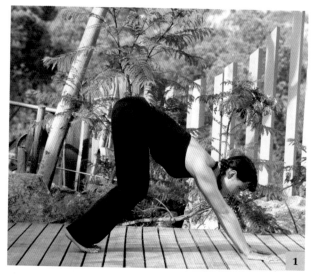

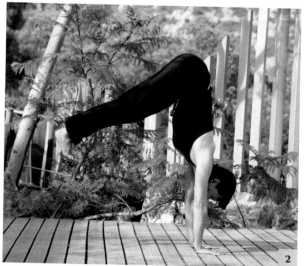

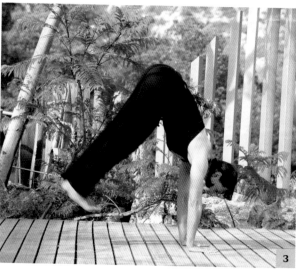

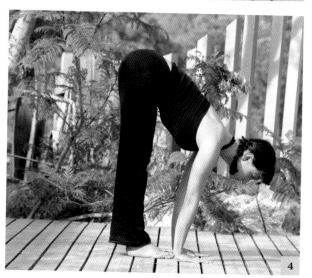

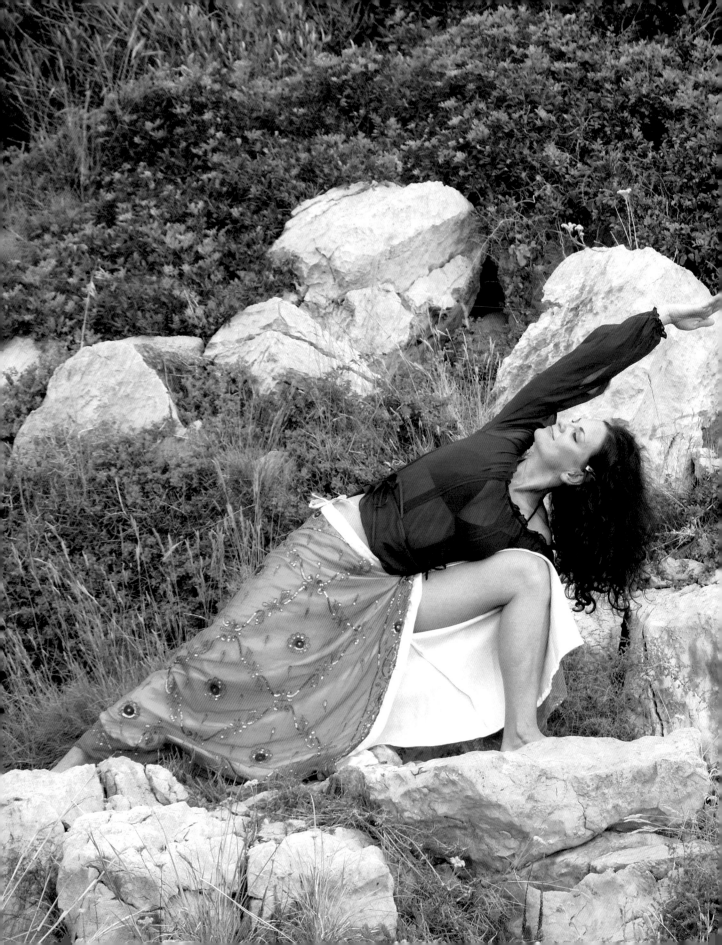

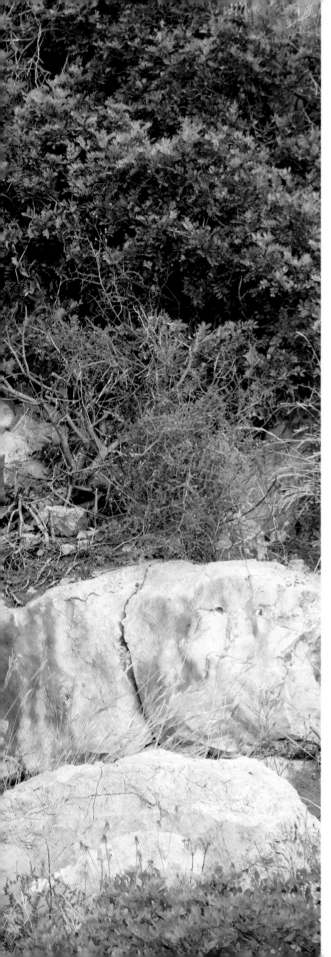

Standing postures

Standing postures are usually practised after the Sun Salutation, when the body is already warmed up. They prepare you for more complicated asanas, generate heat and build up energy.

From a physiological point of view, standing poses strengthen feet and leg muscles and joints. They also strengthen the abdominal muscles and stimulate blood flow. They increase the breathing space and therefore the breathing volume.

On an emotional level, standing postures promote a sense of grounding and stability and therefore a feeling of 'having both feet firmly on the ground'. They also develop stamina and staying power, causing feelings of strength, self-awareness and inner security to grow.

virabhadrasana i **Warrior Pose I**

Warrior Pose I strengthens the leg muscles, ankles and knees. The back muscles are fortified and the neck relaxed. This asana conveys stability and alleviates stiffness in the back.

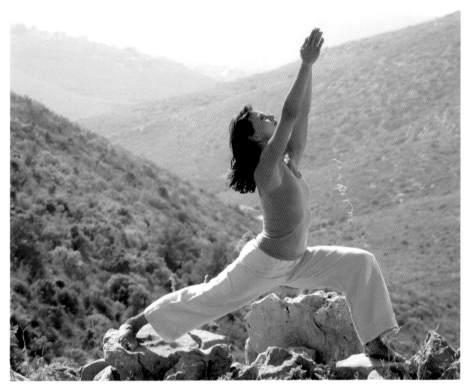

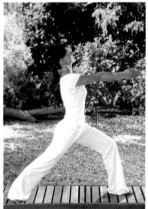

For beginners ▲

Take a smaller step back and lower your arms if you do not feel flexible or strong enough. Make sure your knee remains directly above your ankle.

Alignment

- Take a long step back, placing both heels in a line. Your back foot should be turned in at an angle of about 45 degrees and your front foot should point straight ahead.

- Stretch your back leg and put the weight on the outer edge of this foot, so that the arch of the foot lifts slightly.

- Bend your front leg at right angles and align your knee above your ankle.

- Square your hips, facing forward as far as possible.

- Make sure your chest faces forward and, as you inhale, lengthen up from the thoracic vertebrae.

- On an exhalation, draw your tailbone under and drop deeper into the position.

- Position your shoulders above your hips and lengthen your back still further by gently stretching your arms upwards. Your arms should remain within your field of vision and your shoulders should be relaxed.

- Direct your gaze upwards slightly.

v̄irabhadrās̱ana ïi **Warrior Pose II**

Warrior Pose II strengthens the arm, leg and back muscles as well as the ankles and knees. The hip is opened and the buttocks tensed. The organs of the lower abdomen are also strengthened. The opening of the chest makes it possible to breathe deeply, which helps to increase breathing volume.

Alignment

- Step back as far as you can, placing both heels in a line. Turn your back foot out approximately 90 degrees and point your front foot straight ahead.

- Stretch your back leg and put your weight on the outer edge of your back foot, so that the arch of the foot lifts slightly.

- Bend your front leg at right angles and position your knee above your ankle.

- Open your hips as far as possible and turn both thighs out.

- Align your upper body right over your hips, so that it does not bend forward or back.

- Extend your arms out to shoulder level, keeping your shoulders relaxed. As you inhale, stretch forward and back through your fingertips.

- As you exhale, lower your tailbone and drop your hips deeper into the pose.

- Turn your head in the directon of your front leg and look towards your front hand.

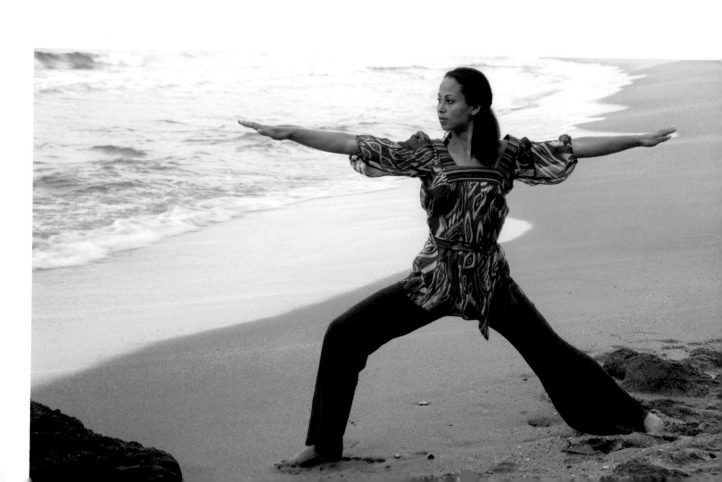

Reverse Warrior Pose

One of the few asanas that have no Sanskrit name, Reverse Warrior Pose, common in yoga practice, strengthens the leg muscles, improves flexibility in the spine, stretches the sides of the upper body and opens the hips.

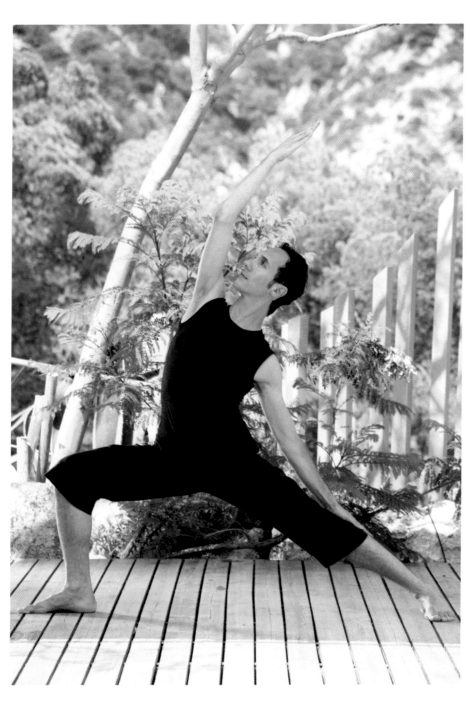

Alignment

- Assume the basic posture of Warrior Pose II (see p.79).

- Raise your front arm so that you feel a pleasant stretch along one side of your body, without buckling on the other side.

- Move the other arm as far as possible down your back leg.

- Inhale and lengthen your spine, exhale and gently lower your hips.

- Bring your gaze slightly upwards.

uｔkaｔaｓaｎa Fierce Pose

In Fierce Pose, the entire upper body is strengthened. The leg muscles and ankles are also strengthened and the calves are stretched. The shoulders remain relaxed. Opening the ribcage stretches the chest muscles and lifting the diaphragm gently massages the heart.

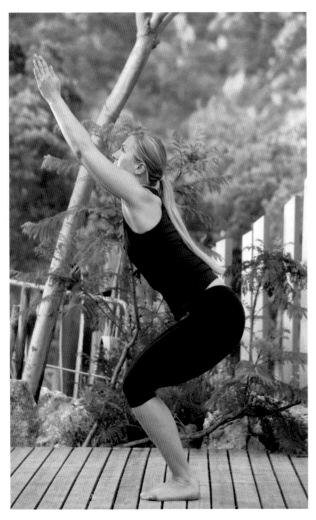

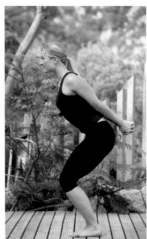

Variation ▲

Clasp your hands behind your back. This will open up your chest further as well as give you a pleasant shoulder stretch.

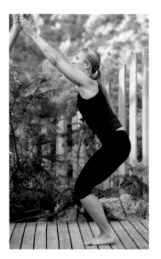

For beginners ▲

Do not bend as low if you feel you lack strength in your thighs.

- Raise your arms and if possible bring your palms together. Turn your upper arms out slightly.

- Draw the crown of your head upwards, tilting your neck back slightly. Look up towards your hands.

- Inhale and lengthen your thoracic vertebrae, pulling your breastbone gently upwards. Your shoulders should remain open and relaxed with the shoulder blades pulled back and lowered softly.

Alignment

- Bend your legs, keeping your knees and ankles together and shifting your weight to the heels. Press your knees together gently, to keep them level. This will also keep your hips parallel.

- As you exhale, lower your tailbone and go deeper into the pose.

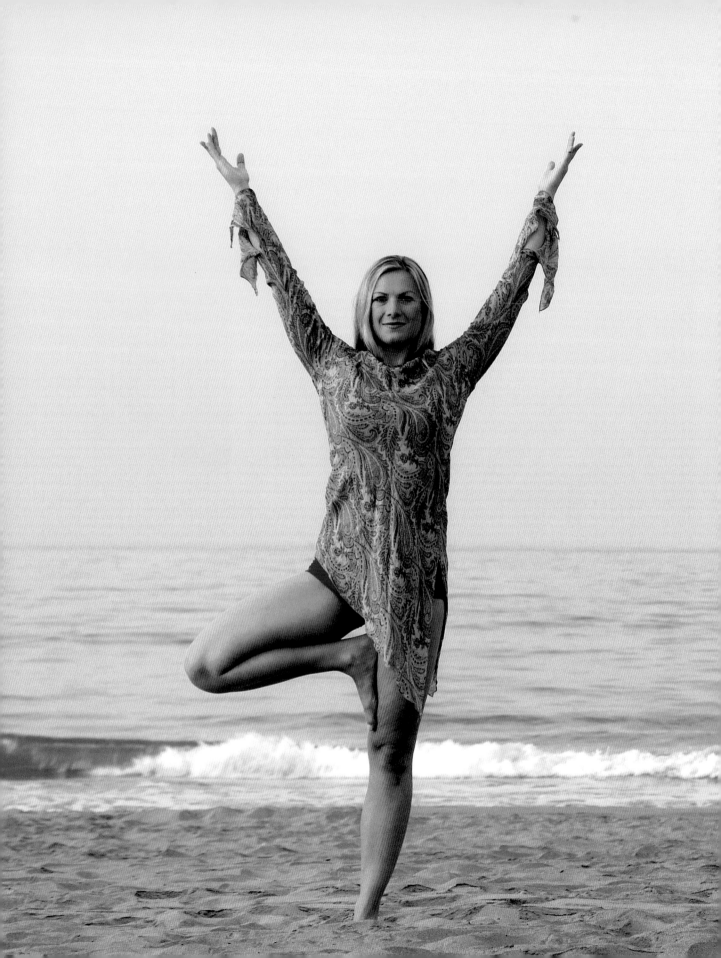

Vriksasana Tree Pose

Apart from the leg muscles, this asana strengthens the muscles and joints of the feet and ankles in particular. It also strengthens the shoulders and back muscles. The hips remain open, which helps promote balance and conveys a feeling of stability and equilibrium.

Alignment

- Find a strong position on your standing leg and put your weight on the whole foot.
- Lift your other leg and place the sole of your foot against the upper inner thigh of the standing leg. Press the sole of your foot firmly against your thigh.
- Extend your arms out to the sides. Keep your shoulders relaxed.
- Inhale and lengthen your spine up through the crown of your head; keep your standing leg pressed firmly into the ground.
- Exhale and draw your tailbone under slightly, while keeping your spine lengthened.

For advanced students ▶

Reach one arm down to your bent leg, while at the same time gently drawing your other arm in to the same side. This stretches the whole side of the body and also promotes a sense of balance. If you are looking for more of a challenge, practise Vriksasana with your eyes closed.

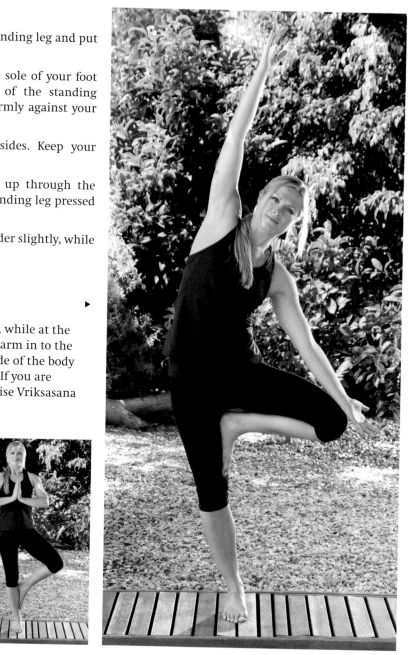

For beginners ▶

If you are not yet able to place the sole of your foot against your upper thigh, place it against your calf but not under any circumstances against the knee. The knee joints are sensitive and you have very little stability in this pose.

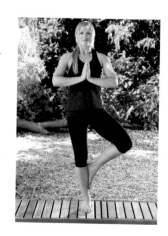

garuḍāsana Eagle Pose

This asana strengthens and stretches the leg and buttock muscles, particularly in the feet and calves. The shoulders are also stretched, and flexibility is increased in the arms and legs. In addition, this asana promotes balance and conveys a feeling of stability and equilibrium.

Alignment

1. Find a stable position on your supporting leg and take the weight through your whole foot. Bend your supporting leg slightly and wrap your other leg around it by positioning the upper thigh on the lower thigh, bringing your knee up as high as possible and twisting your shin behind the calf of your supporting leg. Hook your foot around the calf (see image 1).

2. Straighten your upper body and place the arm on the same side as the twisted leg in the elbow bend of your other arm (see image 2).

3. Wrap your arms around each other, so that you can bring the palms of your hands together with your thumbs pointing towards your face (see image 3).

   - Inhale and lengthen your body upwards through the crown of your head, at the same time pressing your foot firmly into the ground.

   - Exhale and lower your tailbone, while maintaining the length of your spine.

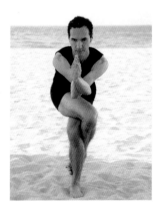

◀ **Variation**

In order to increase the stretch in the shoulders and buttocks, on an inhalation lengthen your body upwards, then on an exhalation bend forward with a long spine.

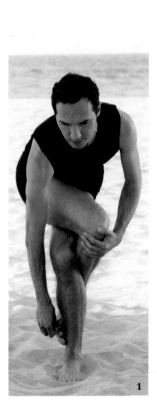

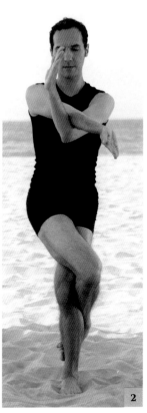

For beginners: if you are not yet able to bring your shin behind your calf, lay your foot on the outside of the supporting leg. If your shoulders are not yet flexible enough, do not bring the palms of your hands together, but position them beneath one another.

For advanced students: practise wrapping both legs and arms around each other at the same time.

1

2

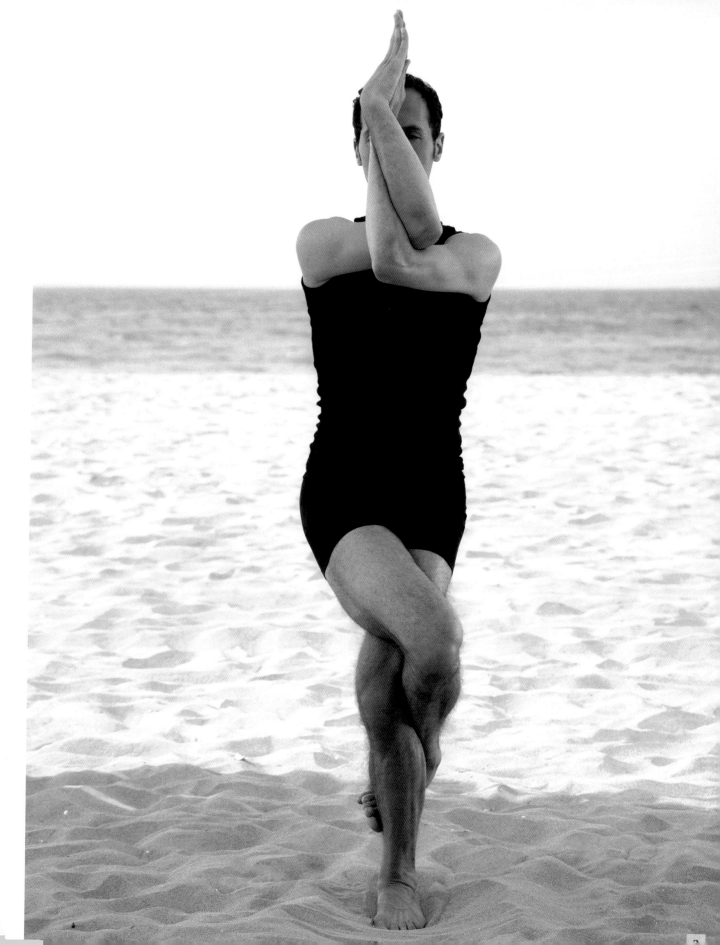

utthita parsvakonasana Extended Side Angle Pose

This asana strengthens the ankles, knees and thighs. At the same time, the side of the body is stretched along its entire length and the hips are opened. This posture improves digestion and alleviates sciatica and arthritis.

Alignment

- Lunge back and turn your back foot to an angle of 90 degrees. Your front foot should be pointing forward.

- Stretch your back leg, taking the weight on the outer edge of the foot, and turn the thigh out slightly.

- Bend your front leg, so that the shin is vertical and the thigh is parallel to the ground.

- Place the hand of your lower arm flat on the ground, on the outer edge of the front foot, and support your weight with the whole of your hand. Your knee should press out towards this arm.

- Stretch your upper arm over your head, lengthening your body diagonally and forward. Your whole body should produce a line from the foot of your straight leg to the fingertips of your hand on the same side. Your weight should be evenly distributed on both legs and the front hand.

- Inhale and stretch from your fingertips to the toes of your back foot.

- Look up and lower your pelvis further into the posture.

For beginners

Rest your lower arm on your thigh and stretch your upper arm over your head, so that your body forms a line. ▼

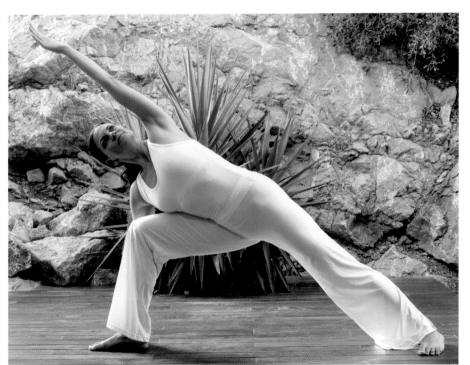

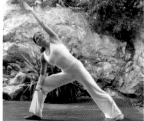

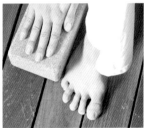

For beginners ▲

If you cannot reach the floor, place a block under your hand.

baddhā parṣvakonasana
Bound Extended Side Angle Pose

This asana has the same effect as Utthita Parsvakonasana. It also includes a shoulder stretch, which opens the shoulders further. This has a positive effect on breathing and improves breathing volume.

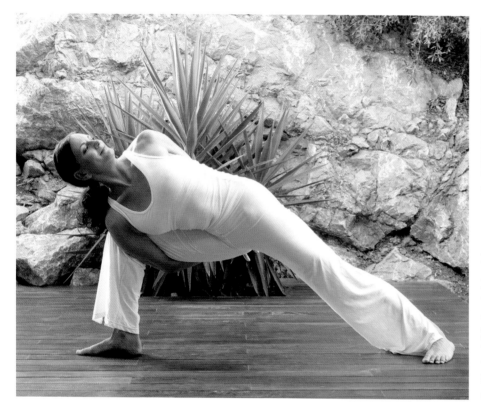

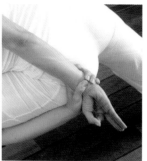

Rear view detail

For beginners

Place your hand flat on the ground to the inside of your front foot, taking your weight through your whole foot. Stretch your upper arm behind your back and place your hand on your bent thigh. ▼

Alignment

- Assume Utthita Parsvakonasana (see p.86).
- From this position, extend your lower arm beneath your bent thigh and take the upper arm behind your back. Grab your fingers or, if possible, the wrist of your upper arm (see rear view detail).
- Exhale and rotate your body to the side, pushing your tailbone back.
- Look up towards the sky.

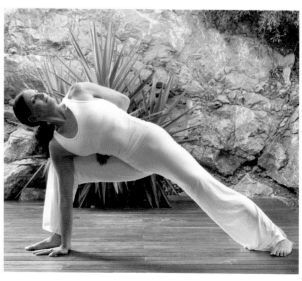

utthita trikonasana Triangle Pose

This asana strengthens the leg muscles and ankles. It also mobilizes the hips and stabilizes the back, helping to alleviate back pain. Triangle Pose can also help relieve tension in the chest, shoulders and pelvis. Opening the chest allows for deeper breathing.

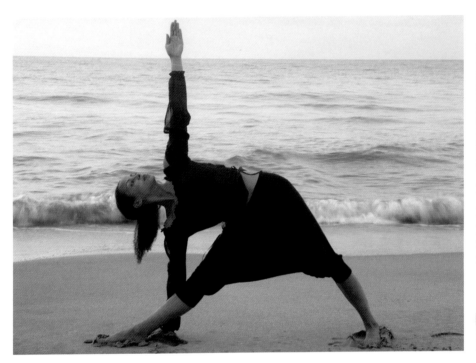

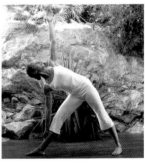

For beginners ▲

Place your hand on your ankle or your calf if you are unable to reach the floor.

If you have neck problems, do not look up but simply down at your front foot.

Alignment

- Step wide apart and position the heels of both feet in a straight line. Turn your front foot forwards and your back foot out by about 45 degrees.

- Draw your kneecaps up gently and turn your front thigh out slightly. Distribute the weight over both legs and press the outer edge of your back foot into the floor.

- Open your hips, with the front hip stretching forward and the back hip stretching back.

- Lift up out of your waist and extend forward over your front leg, placing your hand flat alongside the outer edge of your front foot.

- Stretch your other arm upwards, palm facing forward. Both arms should create a vertical line and your shoulders should remain relaxed.

- Inhale, then twist to the side as you exhale, pushing your lower hip forward and your upper hip back. Push your tailbone back towards the rear heel.

- Your upper body should be stretched on both sides.

- Look up towards your fingertips.

baddha trikonasana **Bound Triangle Pose**

This asana has the same effect as Utthita Trikonasana (opposite). In addition, the shoulders are stretched and the chest is opened up further. This has a positive effect on breathing and improves breathing volume.

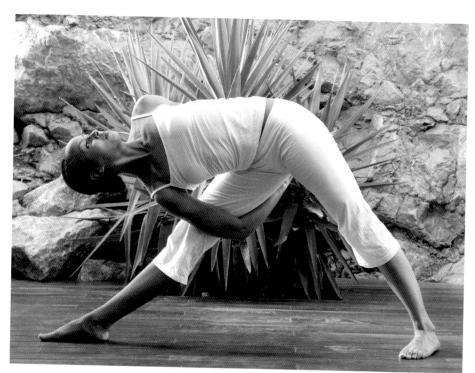

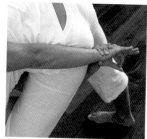

Rear view detail

For beginners

Place your front hand on your calf, take your rear arm behind your back and place your hand on your thigh. ▼

Alignment

- Assume Utthita Trikonasana (see p.88).

- Take your lower arm under your front thigh and your upper arm behind your back. Grab your fingers or, if possible, the wrist of your upper arm (see Rear view detail).

- On the inhalation, stretch forward above the crown of your head and backwards through your back foot.

- On the exhalation, twist the side of your body up further and push your tailbone back.

- Look upwards.

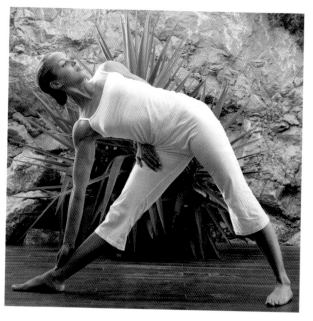

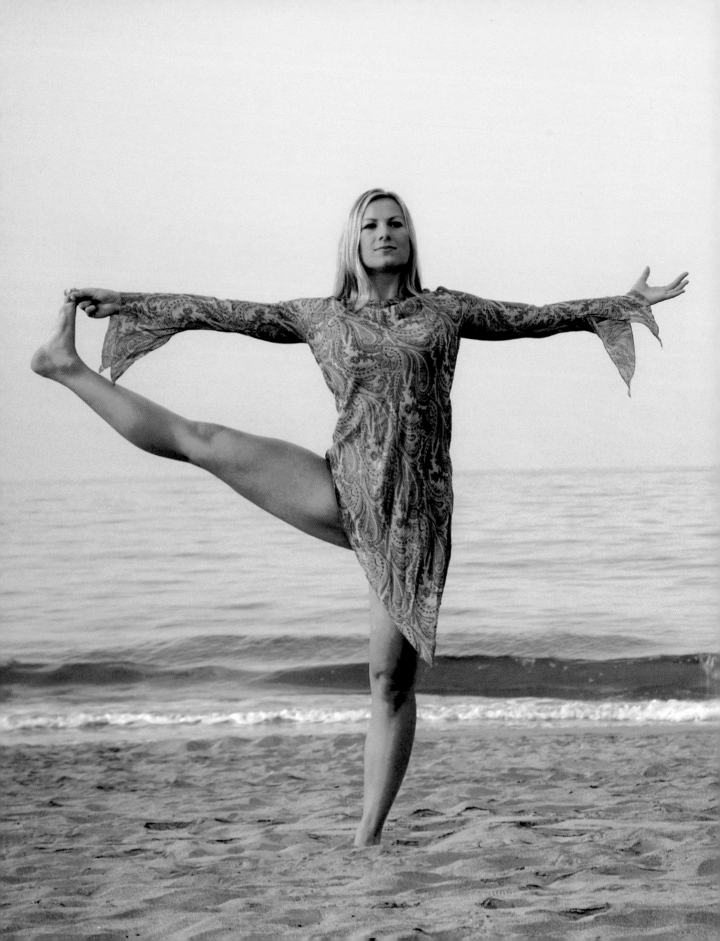

uṫṫhiṫa hasṫa padangusṫhasana
Extended Hand-Toe Pose

This asana strengthens the leg muscles and leg joints, and stretches the hamstrings. The pose also promotes a sense of balance and conveys a feeling of stability and equilibrium.

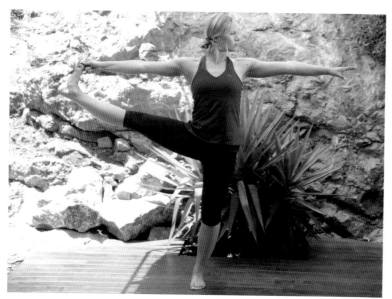

Utthita Hasta Padangusthasana to the side

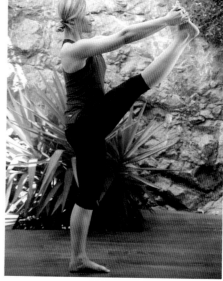

Utthita Hasta Padangusthasana to the front

Alignment

- Find a firm position on your supporting leg and distribute your weight through the entire foot.

- Bend the other leg, grab the big toe or foot and extend the leg out in front of you or to the side.

- The hips should remain parallel.

- On the inhalation, straighten the torso, pull up through the crown of your head and press the foot of your supporting leg firmly into the floor. Lift your chest slightly at the same time.

- On the exhalation, gently pull the leg closer to your body and lower your tailbone.

- Direct your gaze forward or away from your raised leg.

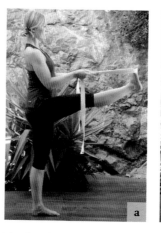

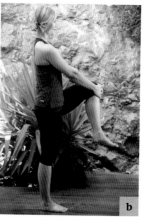

For beginners ▲

a. Use a belt if you cannot grab your foot with your hand. This also helps you to practise the side posture.

b. Bend your raised leg and steady it with both hands. You can also practise this variation to the side.

ardha chandrasana Half Moon Pose

Half Moon Pose strengthens the abdomen, back, buttocks, thighs and ankles. It also strengthens the lumbar vertebrae and the sacrum, and alleviates sciatica. It promotes a sense of balance, creating a feeling of steadiness and stability.

Alignment

- Find a firm position on your supporting leg and distribute your weight over your entire foot. Your foot should be pointing straight in front.

- Place your hand roughly 30cm (12 inches) in front of your supporting foot, lift your other leg up and extend it straight back.

- Straighten your supporting leg and press it firmly into the floor. Straighten your raised leg and push it backwards, making sure your toes are flexed. The foot of your raised leg should be parallel with the floor.

- Open out your hips and turn both thighs out slightly.

- Turn your upper body to the side, forming a line with your straight, raised leg.

- Keep your shoulders relaxed and open as your arms form a vertical line.

- Inhale and stretch forward through the crown of your head and back through your raised foot. Your tailbone should be stretched towards your raised ankle.

- Exhale and twist further to the side, stretching your upper arm gently upwards and your lower arm down. The lower arm should act as a stabilizer but should barely carry any weight.

- Look up towards your extended arm. If you cannot hold your balance, look down.

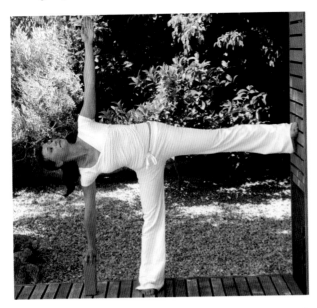

For beginners ▲

Place your lower hand on a block and press the foot of your raised leg firmly against a wall.

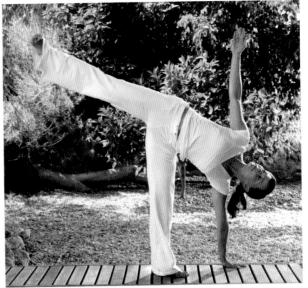

For advanced students ▲

Place your front hand flat on the floor. This will cause your upper body to tilt down further. Extend your raised leg higher, so that your leg and upper body are in line again.

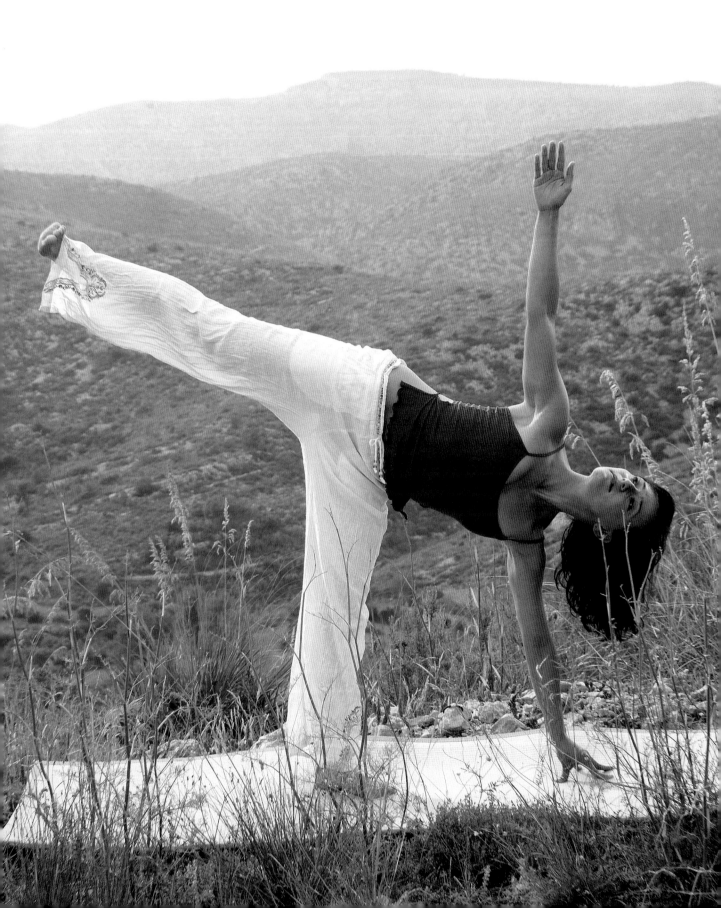

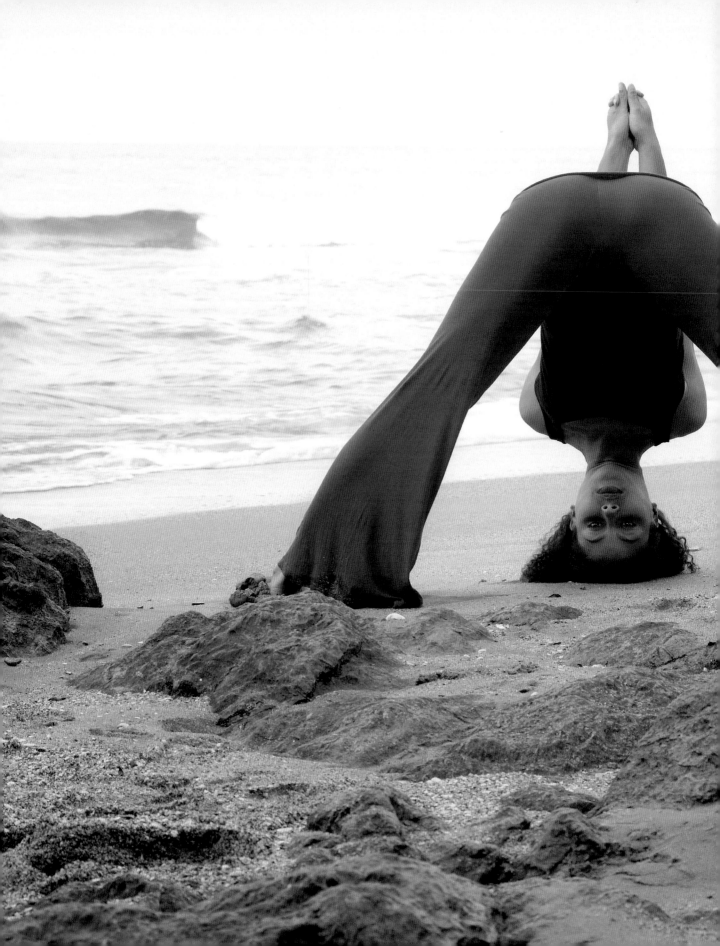

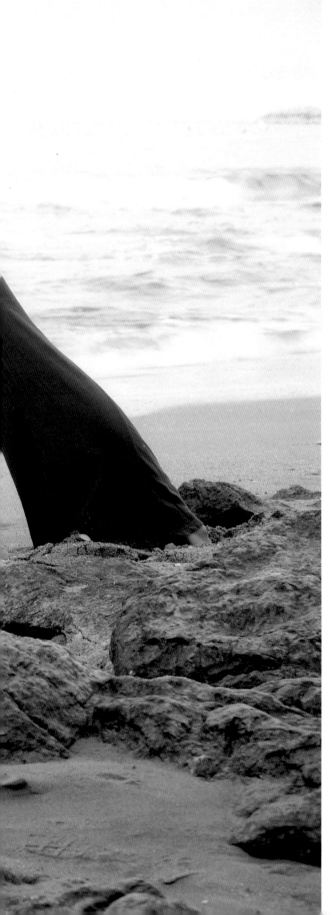

Forward bends

Bending down to pick something up or hunching over to look at a computer screen are familiar actions for many people. Bending forward is therefore a very common everyday posture but it is not particularly good for the back or for a person's sense of well-being. Correctly executed forward bends, on the other hand, benefit the spine.

From a physiological viewpoint, the entire back is stretched, while the fronts of the thighs are taut. Forward bends create space in the waist, the groin, the abdomen and, particularly, the lower back.

On an emotional level, forward bends are above all calming – like a small communion within – and convey the ability to relax and let go. Forward bends are also often accompanied by a look at the past. Emotions can spill over, so that resistance and an impulse to pull out of the forward bend as quickly as possible are felt. Treating yourself with sensitivity and constantly monitoring your breathing help to overcome this resistance and lead to feelings of pure relaxation.

padangusthasana   Hand to Big Toe Pose
padahastasana   Hand to Foot Pose

The effects of these two asanas are the same. The abdominal and digestive organs are strengthened, alleviating gastro-intestinal complaints, and the lumbar vertebrae and sacrum are relaxed, which can alleviate back pain. Both postures have a calming, relaxing effect, with Padahastasana involving a slightly deeper forward bend.

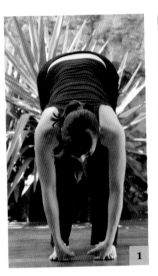 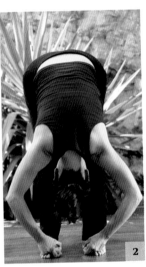

◄ **Padangusthasana**

Step-by-step alignment

1. Bend forward from a standing position and grip your big toes with your index and middle fingers. Inhale and stretch forward from your lower back through the crown of your head and push your tailbone up.

2. Exhale and bend from your hips further towards your legs. Bend your arms out and draw your upper body as close as possible to your thighs. Bring your gaze towards your legs.

Padahastasana   ▶

Step-by-step alignment

1. Bend forward from a standing position. Bend your legs and place your hands under your feet. Inhale and stretch forward from the lower back through the crown of your head and push your tailbone up.

2. Exhale and bend from the hips further towards your legs. Straighten your legs and draw your upper body as close as possible to your thighs. Bring your gaze towards your legs.

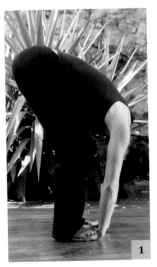 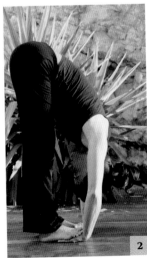

eka pada adho mukha svanasana
One Leg Downward Facing Dog Pose

This asana strengthens all the muscles in the arms, legs and buttocks. At the same time, the backs of the thighs and the calves are stretched alternately. The asana also relieves stress on the back. The shoulder and neck muscles should remain relaxed. The posture requires a good sense of balance and a degree of strength.

Alignment

- Go into Adho Mukha Svanasana (see p.67). Stretch one leg straight up, keeping your hips parallel and facing forward.

- Inhale and stretch through your raised foot and up through the crown of your head. As you exhale, press your hands into the ground, at the same time 'pushing' the floor away from you.

- Bring your gaze down to the floor.

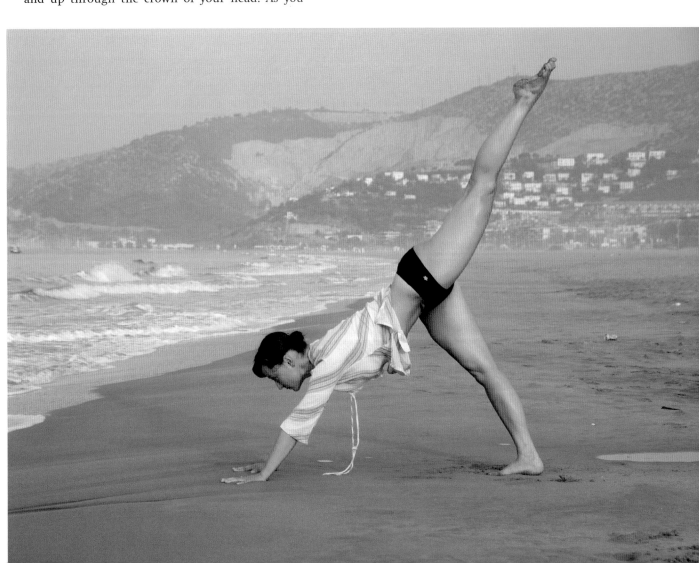

पार्श्वोत्तानासन parsvottanasana Intense Side Stretch Pose

This asana strengthens the fronts of the legs and gives the backs of the legs an intense stretch. It also relaxes any stiffness in the legs, hip muscles and joints and has a relaxing effect on the back as a whole.

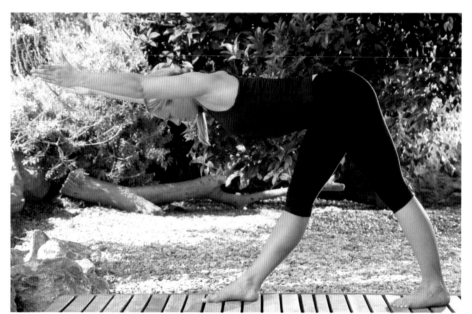

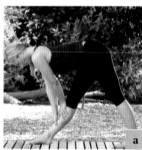

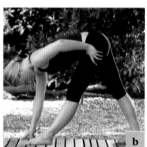

Starting posture ▲

Alignment

- Step out about 1 metre (3 feet) to the side, keeping both feet and your hips forward. Your leg muscles should remain stretched.

- Exhale and bend forward from your waist. Inhale and extend your arms forward, stretching from your lower back while drawing forward through the crown of your head. Raise your sternum up slightly and push your tailbone back (see Starting posture).

- Exhale and bend further from your hips towards your thighs, pushing your tailbone and sit bones upwards.

- Place your hands in the prayer position (Namaste) against your back (see p.53) or grip your elbows if this is too difficult.

- Move your nose towards your knee and relax your neck. Look towards your leg.

Vary the length of your step, in order to achieve an intense but at the same time comfortable stretch.

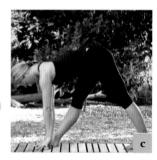

For beginners

a. Place your hands on your shin and practise bending forward from your lower back.

b. Once you have mastered Variant (a), place your hand opposite your front leg on the floor and gently push back your front hip with the other hand.

c. Alternatively, place both hands on the floor; if you are able to, keep your back straight while doing this.

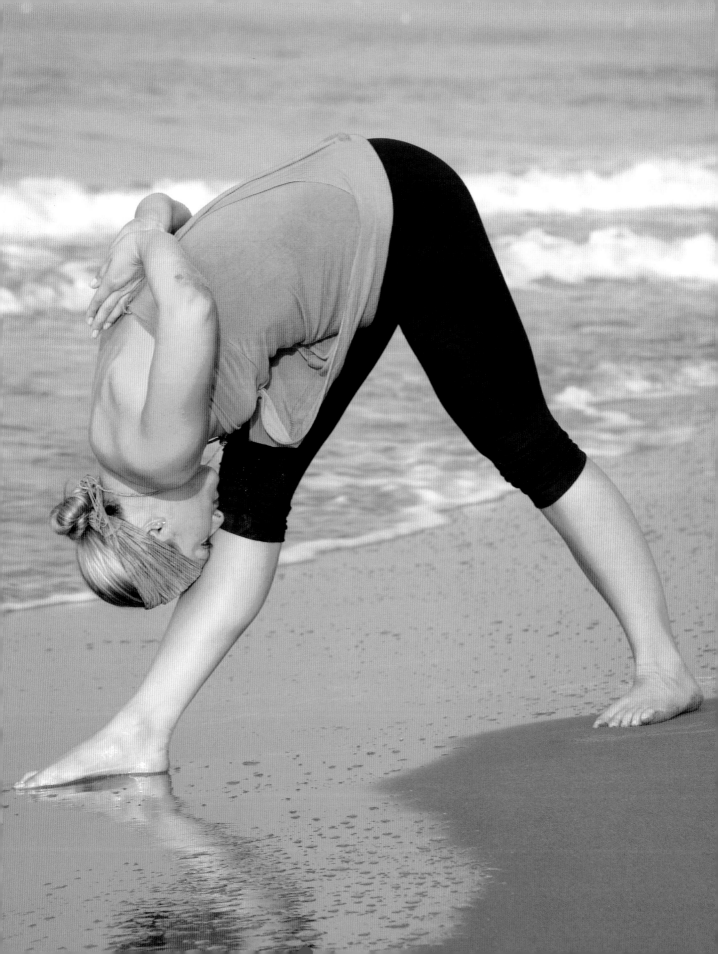

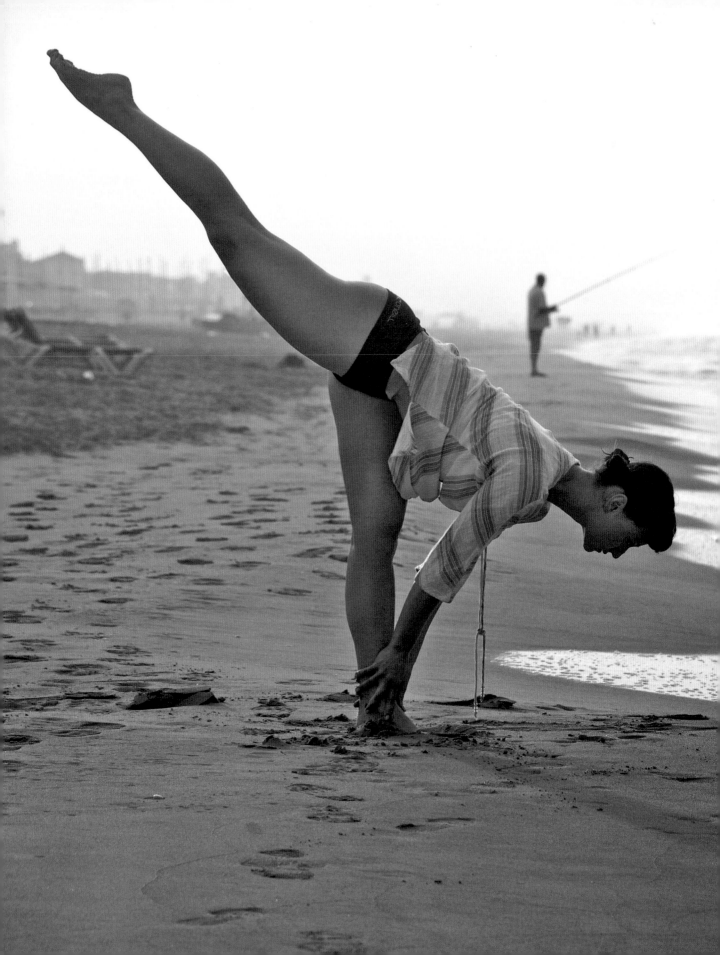

urdhva prasarita ekapadasana
One Foot Extended Upwards Pose

This asana strengthens the foot and leg muscles as well as the buttocks. At the same time, both the fronts and backs of the thighs are alternately stretched intensely. The shoulder and neck muscles remain relaxed. Although this posture requires a good sense of balance and strength in the legs, overall it relieves stress on the back.

Alignment

- Find a comfortable position on your standing leg. Exhale and bend forward, stretching one leg back as high and as straight as possible. The hips should remain parallel and should point forward. Take both hands to the foot of your standing leg with your arms stretched.

- On an inhalation, lengthen your lower back, pull forward through the crown of your head and up through the heels of your raised leg.

- On an exhalation, bend further forward from your hips and bring your upper body as close as possible to the thigh of your standing leg.

- Bring your gaze down.

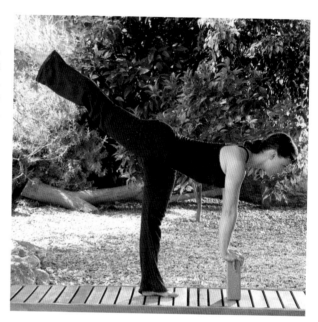

For beginners ▲

Place your hands on a block in front of you, parallel to your shoulders. If you want to go further, place both hands on the floor, then try to take one hand to the foot of your standing leg, while you balance yourself with your other hand.

◄ For advanced students

a. Raise your back leg higher and bring your upper body as close as possible to the thigh of your standing leg, until your nose touches your standing leg. Keep this leg straight. Look towards your standing leg.

b. To intensify the stretch on the front and back of your thigh, you can also practise this pose against a wall, to develop a feeling of when your legs are in a vertical line. Bring your gaze to your standing leg.

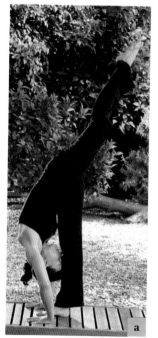

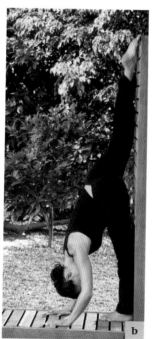

praṣarita padottanaṣana
Wide Leg Forward Bend

This asana strengthens the front and outer thigh muscles. The inner thigh muscles and hamstrings are also given an intense stretch and the knee muscles are strengthened. The digestive organs are stimulated, regulating digestion, and the whole back is relieved of stress.

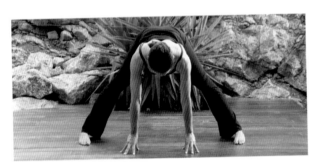

Starting posture

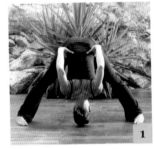

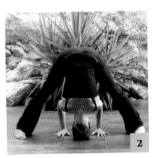

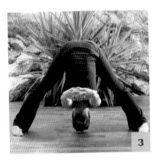

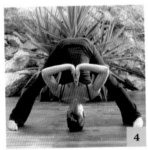

> If you can rest your head on the floor easily, reduce the gap between your feet. Because the head carries no weight in this asana, you can try this posture as an alternative to the headstand, especially if you have neck problems and are unable to perform the headstand.

Alignment

- Go into this forward bend by placing your legs wide apart and your feet parallel, turning your big toes in slightly.

- As you exhale, bend forward with a straight back and place your hands on the floor directly below your shoulders. Both your legs should remain stretched (see Starting posture).

- Inhale and lengthen up through your spine.

- As you exhale, bend forward from your hips. Ease the crown of your head down towards the floor and lift your tailbone and sit bones upwards.

- Make sure your breathing remains even throughout the different arm postures.

Cycle of different arm postures

1. Place your hands on your hips, thereby supporting the bend from your hips.

2. Move your hands back between your feet, bending your elbows.

3. Fold your hands behind your back and stretch your arms forward, parallel to the floor.

4. Bring your hands into the prayer position (Namaste, see p.53) against your back.

5. Grip each ankle with your hands.

Your neck should remain relaxed in each of these postures and should not bear any weight.

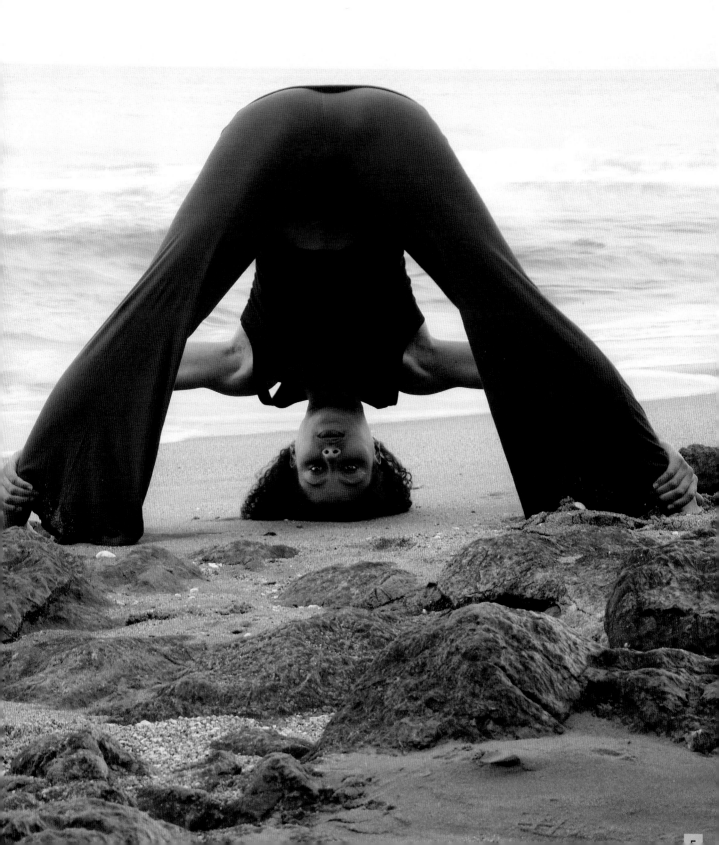

ꡲomukhaṣana Cow Face Pose

In this posture, the hips, legs and knees in particular become supple and flexible. At the same time, the shoulders are stretched intensely and opened. The chest cavity is expanded and the whole spine is stretched.

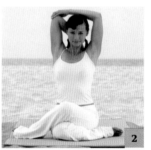
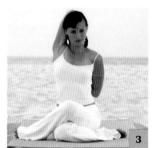

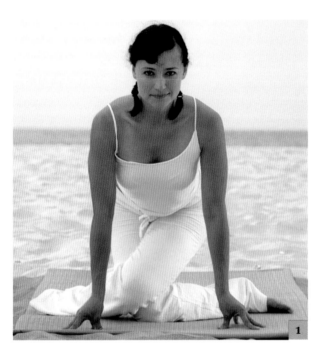

Step-by-step alignment

1. Get onto all fours and cross your legs so that one knee is exactly in front of the other. The sides of your feet should rest on the floor.

2. Lower your buttocks to the floor between your feet and bend the arm opposite the upper knee so far behind your body that the palm of your hand reaches between your shoulders. Gently push your elbow back with your other hand.

3. Bring your other arm up behind your body and grip the fingertips or wrist of your upper arm. As you inhale, draw yourself up from the spine through the crown of your head.

4. As you exhale, bend forward from your hips and push your tailbone down. Your back should remain straight. Gently press your head against your arm to keep your shoulders open.

For beginners ▼

a. Place a cushion between your knees or sit on a block if you cannot yet sit comfortably between your feet in this position.

b. If you cannot yet bring your hands together behind your back, use a belt.

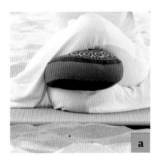
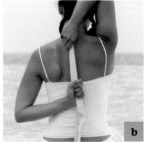

Forward bends

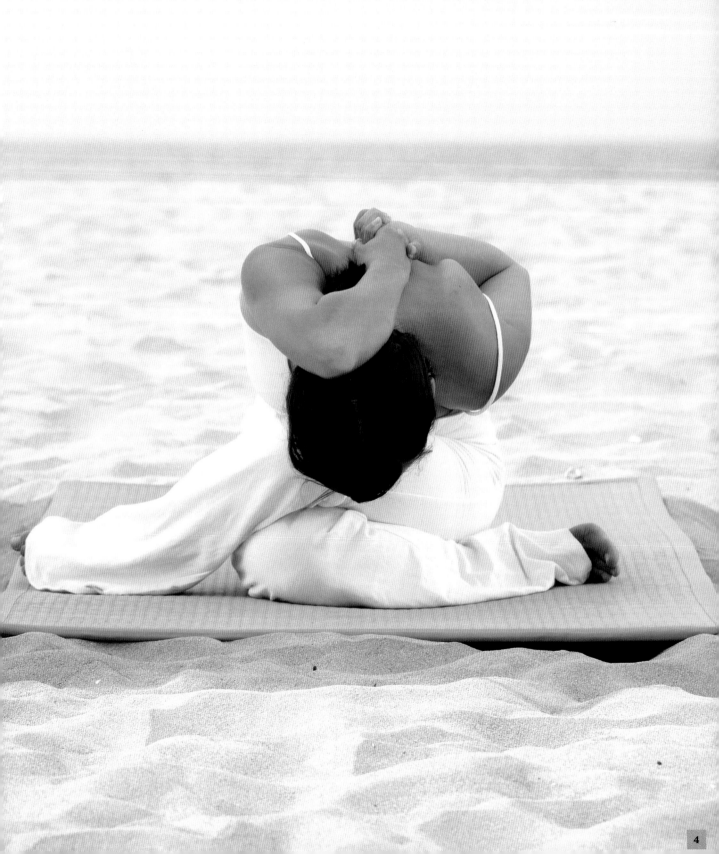

baddha konasana Bound Angle Pose

This asana stretches the pelvis, stomach, buttocks and back (particularly the lower region). Kidney, prostate and bladder function are also stimulated, so that urinary tract conditions may be alleviated. Bound Angle Pose promotes regular menstruation in women.

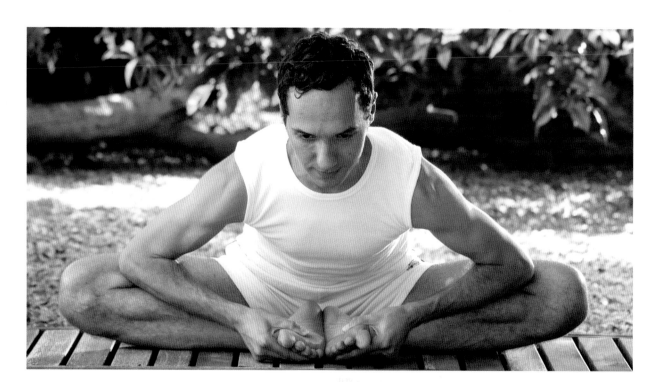

Alignment

- Sit upright and pull your knees in towards your chest. Allow your knees to drop to the sides and pull your heels in as close as possible to your pubic bone.

- Turn the soles of your feet upwards and gently press your arms against your thighs to open your hips out further. Your thighs should be drawn out and down.

- As you inhale, draw your spine up through the crown of your head.

- Exhale and bend forward from your hips, pushing your tailbone back. Draw your navel towards your feet and gently press your knees further down to the floor with your elbows.

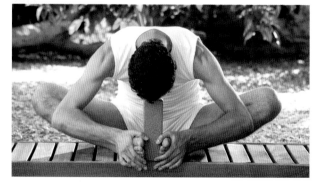

For beginners ▲

Place a block between your feet and rest your head on it. You can also place cushions under your knees or sit on a block or a cushion.

द्वि पादा राजकपोतासन **Double Pigeon Pose**

This asana has the same effect as Baddha Konasana (opposite). It opens and stretches the hips and knees, but even more intensely. With a little practice, this asana can be used to solve stubborn tensions in the buttocks.

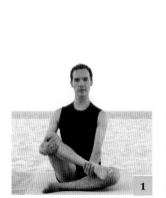
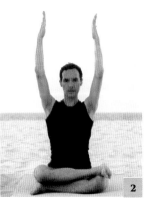

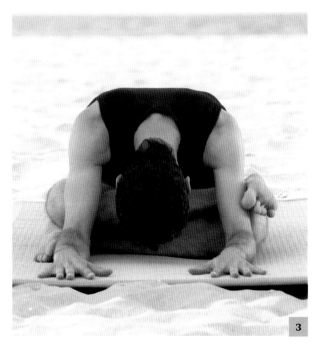

Step-by-step alignment

1. Get into a seated position. Bend one leg and position it so that your shin bone is parallel to the floor in front of you. Bend your other leg and rest the knee on the ankle of your lower foot and place the upper ankle on the knee of your lower leg.

2. As you inhale, stretch your arms upwards and pull your spine up through the crown of your head.

3. Exhale and bend from the hips as far forward as you can, pushing your tailbone back at the same time. Your back should remain straight. Place your arms in front of you and relax your neck.

• Keep your breathing even and try to relax your hips as far as possible.

▼ For beginners

a. If you find that you cannot open your hips very far, lay your shin bones one in front of the other.

b. Alternatively, stretch one leg out, bend your other leg and lay the outer ankle bone on the lower knee.

c. If you cannot lower your knee to your inside ankle bone, place a cushion between your knee and your ankle bone.

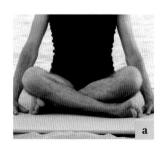
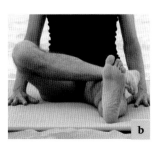
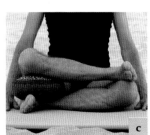

Make sure your shins are straight in front of you and lie parallel on top of each other.

Forward bends

upavishtha konasana Seated Angle Pose

This asana strengthens the front and back thigh muscles. The inner and back thigh muscles are also given an intense stretch and the knee muscles are strengthened. Blood flows to the pelvis, which can alleviate sciatica and menstrual problems.

Forward bends

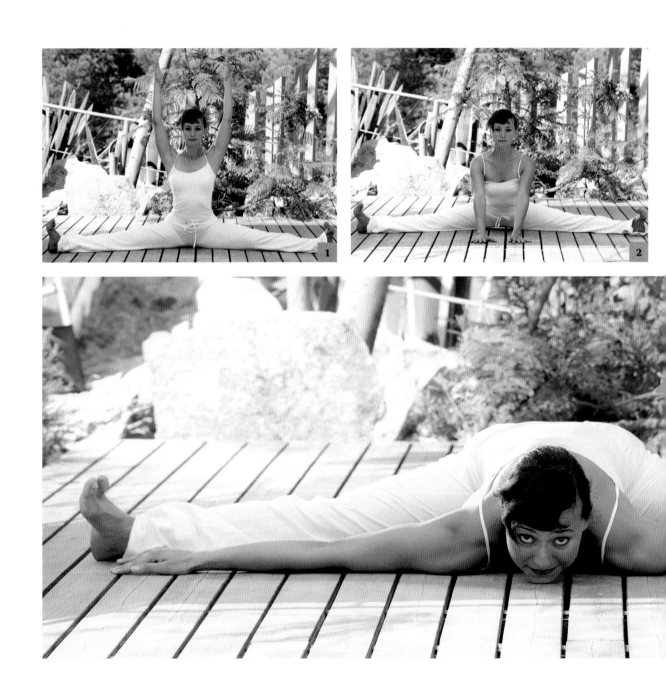

For beginners

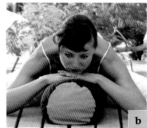

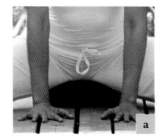

a. Sit on a cushion so that the pelvis is straight. Bending your legs slightly will make this even easier.

b. Place a cushion in front of you and lower your torso onto it if you are not yet able to lower your chin to the floor.

c. Only bend as far forward as you can while keeping your back straight.

Step-by-step alignment

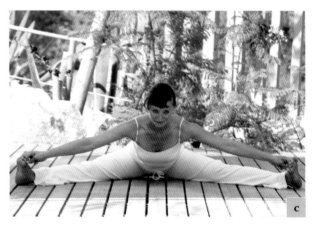

1. Sit with your legs spread out wide, tensing your leg muscles. As you inhale, stretch your arms up, lengthening your spine through the crown of your head. Your pelvis and back should be straight.

2. Exhale and bend forward as far as possible with a straight back and press your hands down into the floor. Keep pushing your tailbone back.

3. As you inhale, lengthen your torso again, then exhale and lower your chin to the floor. Keep your back straight and stretch your arms out parallel to your legs.

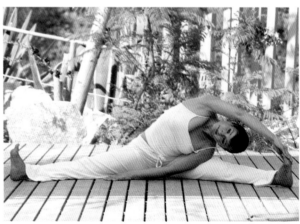

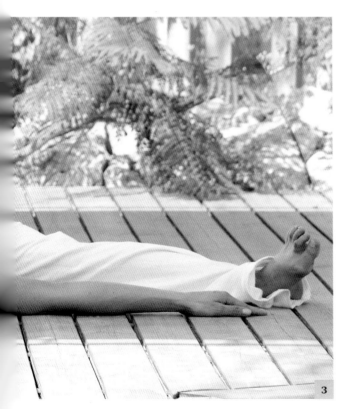

Variation

As you inhale, bring your shoulder as close as possible to your knee and turn to the side as you exhale. Grab your toe with your other hand. This variation is a side bend and gives the side of the body an intense stretch.

Forward bends

pashchimottanasana   Intense West Stretch Pose

This asana stretches the whole of the back as well as the hamstrings and buttock muscles. The abdominal organs are strengthened and digestion is regulated. The spine is strengthened by the stretch and the heart is massaged, so that the pose has both a calming and an energizing effect.

Alignment

- Sit upright with your legs stretched out in front of you. Tense your legs keeping your feet flexed and as you inhale stretch your arms upwards. Lengthen your spine through the crown of your head. Your pelvis should be straight and your back upright.

- As you exhale, bend forward from your hips while pushing your tailbone back. Your back, particularly your lower back, should remain as straight as possible.

- Grip the outsides of your feet and gently pull them out. Your thumb should press on the knuckle of your big toe. Alternatively, place a yoga block behind your feet and grip it with your hands. Lower your torso onto your thighs, relax your neck and gently draw your head to your legs.

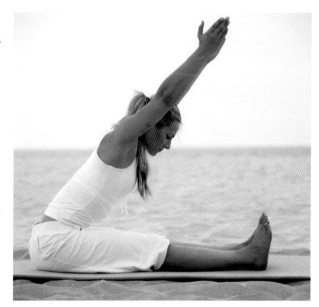

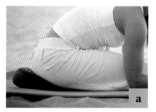

For beginners ▶

a. Sit on a cushion if you are unable to straighten your pelvis. If necessary, bend your legs too.

b. Use a belt if you cannot grab your feet with your hands.

c. Use a cushion for your head to rest on if you cannot bring it to your legs.

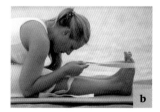

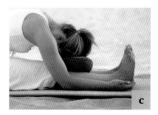

ēka pāda rājakapotāsana
One-Legged King Pigeon Variation

This asana opens the hips and stretches the front thigh muscles and the hip flexor. The abdominal organs are also gently massaged. Overall, this posture has a calming effect, despite the intensive stretch, and has a devotional aspect to it.

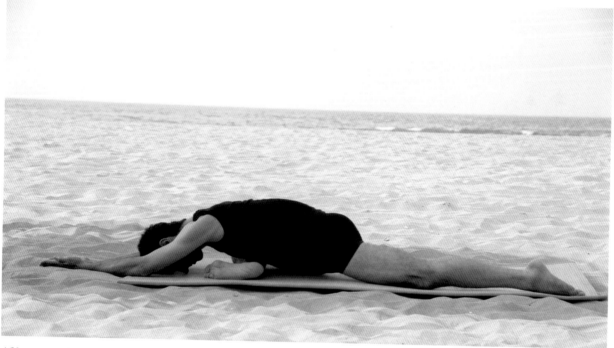

Alignment

- Sit up straight with your legs bent and stretch one leg out behind you with the sole of your foot facing up. Bend your front leg into a right angle, keeping the sole of this foot facing upwards. Both hips should be on the floor.

- Place your hands alongside your hips, press them into the ground as you inhale and lengthen your spine through the crown of your head (see Starting posture).

- Exhale and bend forward with a straight back, pushing your tailbone back. Rest your forehead on the floor and stretch your arms forward with your palms facing upwards.

For beginners

If the hip of your front leg lifts off the floor, place a cushion under it, so that your hips remain parallel.

▼

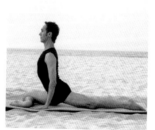

Starting posture

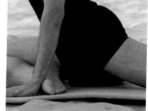

मारिच्यासन अ Marichi's Pose A

This asana, named after the sage Marichi, stretches the shoulders, hamstrings and buttocks. The abdominal organs are constricted, which massages them and stimulates their blood flow. The lower back is strengthened and the upper back and neck muscles relaxed.

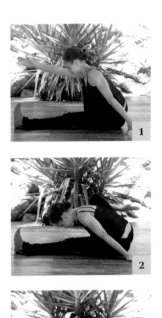

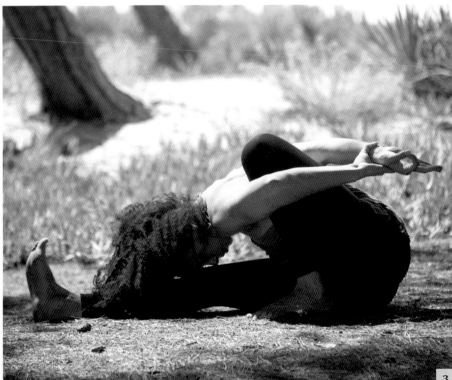

View from opposite side

Step-by-step alignment

1. Sit upright with your legs outstretched. Bend one leg and place your foot a hand-width from the top of your outstretched leg as close as possible to your buttocks. Your outstretched leg should remain tensed. As you inhale, stretch your opposite arm forward towards your foot and lengthen your spine.

2. Exhale and wrap this arm around your bent knee, taking it behind your back. Inhale and lengthen your body again.

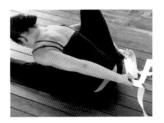

◄ For beginners

If you cannot bring your hands together behind your back, use a belt.

3. As you exhale, take your other arm behind your back and bring your hands together. Bend forward from your hips towards your bent knee, keeping your lower back straight.

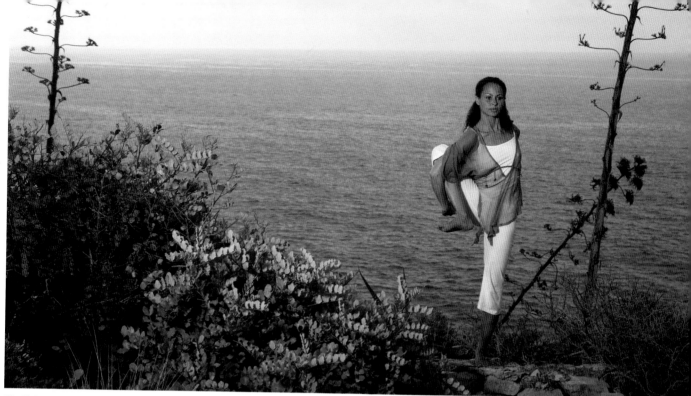

Marichi's Pose A – Standing Variation

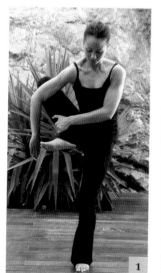

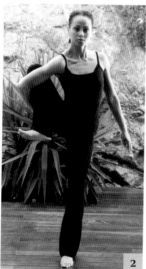

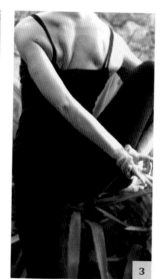

View from behind

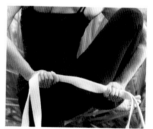

For beginners ▲

If you cannot bring your hands together behind your back, use a belt.

> Marichi's Pose A – Standing Variation is not a forward bend in the true sense, but is included here because it is based on Marichi's Pose A.

Marichi's Pose A – Standing Variation

Step-by-step alignment

1. Find a firm position on your standing leg. Inhale and bend one knee, drawing it up as high as possible alongside your torso.

2. As you exhale, wrap the arm of the same side around your raised knee towards your back. Inhale and press your standing foot into the ground while lengthening your spine through the crown of your head.

3. Exhale and take your other arm behind your back to bring your hands together.

supta padangusthasana Reclining Big Toe Pose

This asana stretches the backs and sides of the legs and the muscles of the buttocks. It can alleviate complaints such as sciatica and stiffness in the legs and hips. The lower back is released, which has a positive effect on back pain.

Alignment

- Lie flat on your back. As you inhale, raise one leg and grab your foot or big toe.
- Tense the muscles in both legs and stretch your raised leg as you exhale and gently draw it as close as possible to your body. Flex the foot and push the heels back or up.
- The entire back, particularly the lower back, shoulders and head should remain on the ground.
- Direct your gaze diagonally upwards.

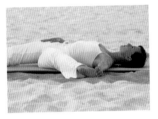

Side variation ▲

As you exhale, allow your raised leg to drop out to the side while keeping your hip on the floor.

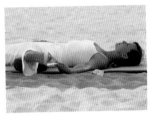

Side variation for beginners ▲

Use a belt and steady your outstretched leg with a cushion if you cannot lower it to the floor.

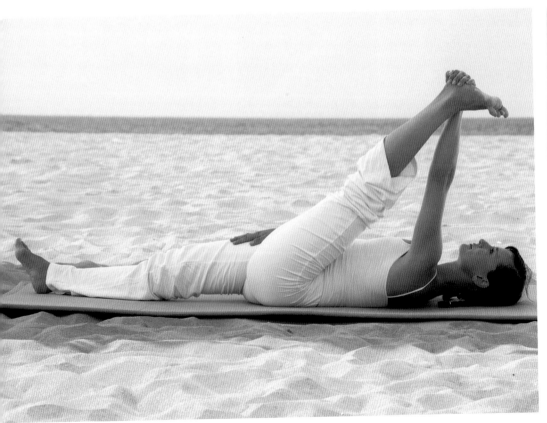

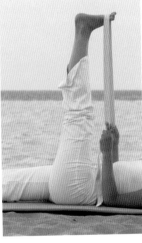

For beginners ▲

Use a belt if you cannot stretch your leg upwards. Rest both elbows on the ground while doing this.

◀ *Leg stretched above in Supta Padangusthasana*

jʌnu shirshʌsʌnʌ Head to Knee Pose

This asana gives an intense stretch to the hamstrings and opens up the hips. The abdominal and digestive organs are massaged, which stimulates digestion. The back and neck muscles are released.

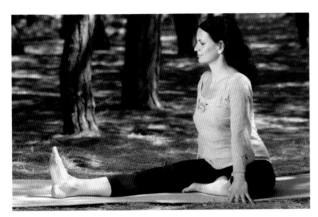

Starting posture

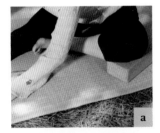

◄ For beginners

a. Place a block under your bent knee if it will not reach the floor.

Alignment

- Sit on the floor with your back straight and bend one leg to the side. Lay your foot on the inside of your outstretched leg, as close as possible to your pubic bone.

- Tense your outstretched leg and push forward through your flexed foot. As you inhale, lengthen from your lower back through the crown of your head (see Starting posture).

- As you exhale, turn slightly towards your outstretched leg and bend forward from your hips, keeping your lower back straight.

- At the same time, push your tailbone back and bring your chest as close as possible to your thigh.

- Place both hands on or around your outstretched foot and rest your head on your knee.

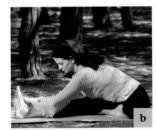

For beginners ▲

b. Only bend forward as far as you can while keeping your back straight. Take hold of the outside of your front foot and gently pull yourself towards your knee. Steady yourself by placing your other hand on the floor.

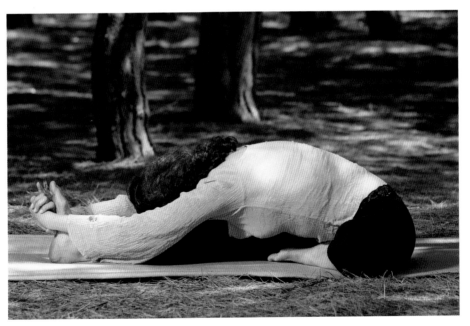

triang mukhaikapada pashchimottanasana
Three Limbs Facing Intense West Stretch Pose

This asana stretches the entire back of the body; at the same time, the ankles and knees are loosened and the abdominal organs are massaged. This posture promotes overall flexibility throughout the body and dispels any feelings of stiffness and apathy.

Alignment

- Sit upright on the floor and bend one leg into Virasana (see p.204). Tense your outstretched leg, flex your foot and push it forward.

- As you inhale, stretch your hands above your head and extend up from your lower back through the crown of your head.

- Exhale and bend forward from your hips over your outstretched leg, keeping your lower back straight. Push your tailbone back at the same time. Bring your chest as close as possible to your outstretched leg.

- Clasp your hands around your foot or grab hold of your wrist and bring your head to your knee.

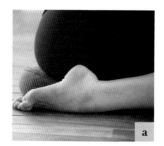

◄ **For beginners**

a. If you find Virasana uncomfortable, place a cushion under your hips.

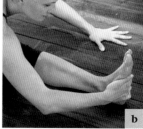

For beginners ▲

b. If your hips are not parallel, grab the foot of your outstretched leg with one arm and place your other hand to the side of your outstretched leg.

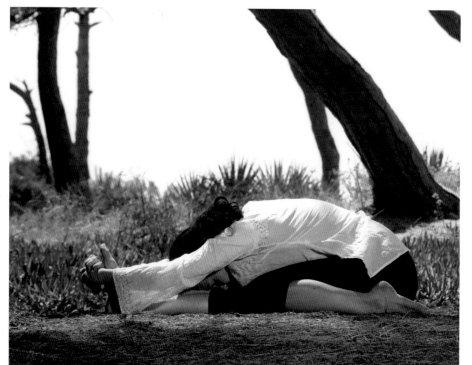

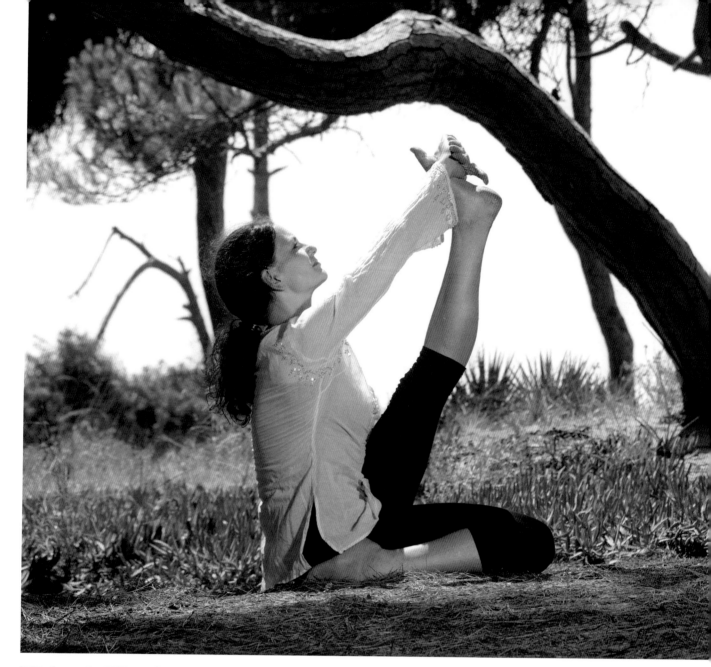

Upward variation ▲

Remain sitting upright, raise your outstretched leg
and pull it in as close as possible to your chest.
Your pelvis and back should remain straight.

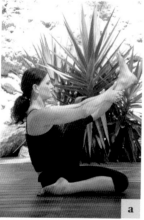
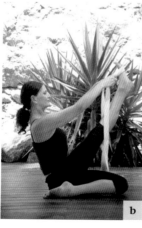

◄ **For beginners**

a. Bend your outstretched leg and grip your calf or
    ankle, if you are not yet able to stretch your leg
    while maintaining a straight back.

b. Use a belt to gently coax your leg into a stretch.

ardha baddha padmottanasana
Half Bound Lotus Standing Forward Bend

This asana stretches the entire back of the body. At the same time, the ankles, knees, shoulder joints and wrists are loosened and the abdominal organs are massaged. This posture promotes flexibility throughout the body and gets rid of stiffness and apathy. The sense of balance is also tested.

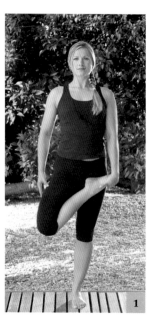
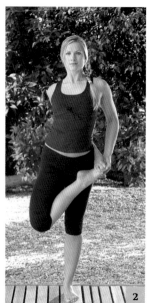
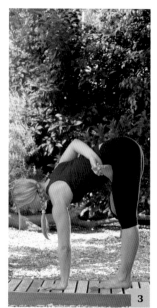
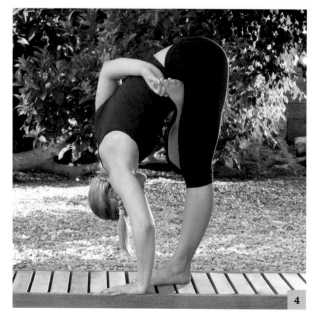

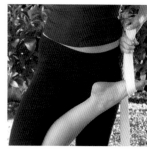

For beginners ▲

Use a belt if you cannot grip your toes in Half Lotus pose.

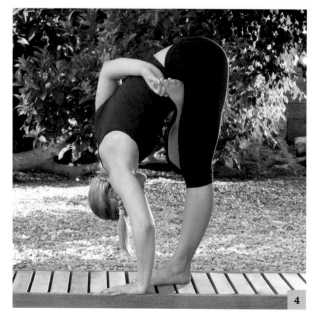

Step-by-step alignment

1. Find your balance and tense your standing leg while placing your other leg in Ardha Padmasana (see p.206). Use your hand to steady your foot in Ardha Padmasana.

2. As you inhale, take your other hand behind your back and grip the toes of your foot.

3. Exhale and bend forward, placing your front hand flat on the ground. Inhale and lengthen through your spine.

4. As you exhale, bend as far forward as possible from your lower back while pushing your tailbone and sit bones back. Release your neck and upper back.

ardha baddha padma pashchimottanasana
Half Bound Lotus Seated Forward Bend

In this asana, the entire back of the body is stretched. At the same time, the ankles, knees, shoulder joints and wrists are loosened and the abdominal organs are massaged. This posture promotes flexibility throughout the whole body and gets rid of feelings of stiffness and apathy.

Step-by-step alignment

1. Sit up with a straight back and place one leg in Ardha Padmasana (see p.206). Tense your outstretched leg and bring the flexed foot of your bent leg gently in towards your body.

2. Steady yourself with one hand. As you inhale, take your other hand behind your back and grip the toes of your bent leg. Lengthen your spine through the crown of your head.

3. Exhale and bend forward from your lower back as far as possible over your outstretched leg and grip the outside of the foot of your outstretched leg. At the same time, push your tailbone back. Release your neck and upper back and lay your head on your outstretched leg.

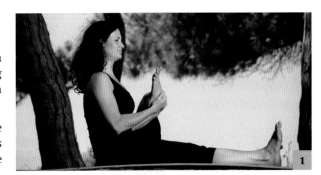

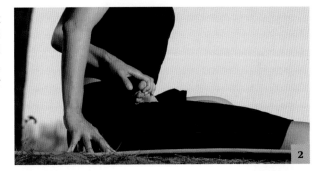

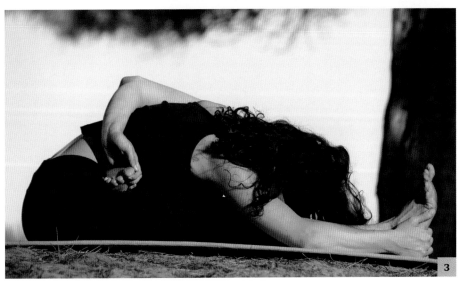

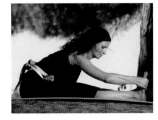

For beginners ▲

Use a belt if you are unable to grip the toes of your bent leg. Only bend as far forward as you can while keeping your lower back straight.

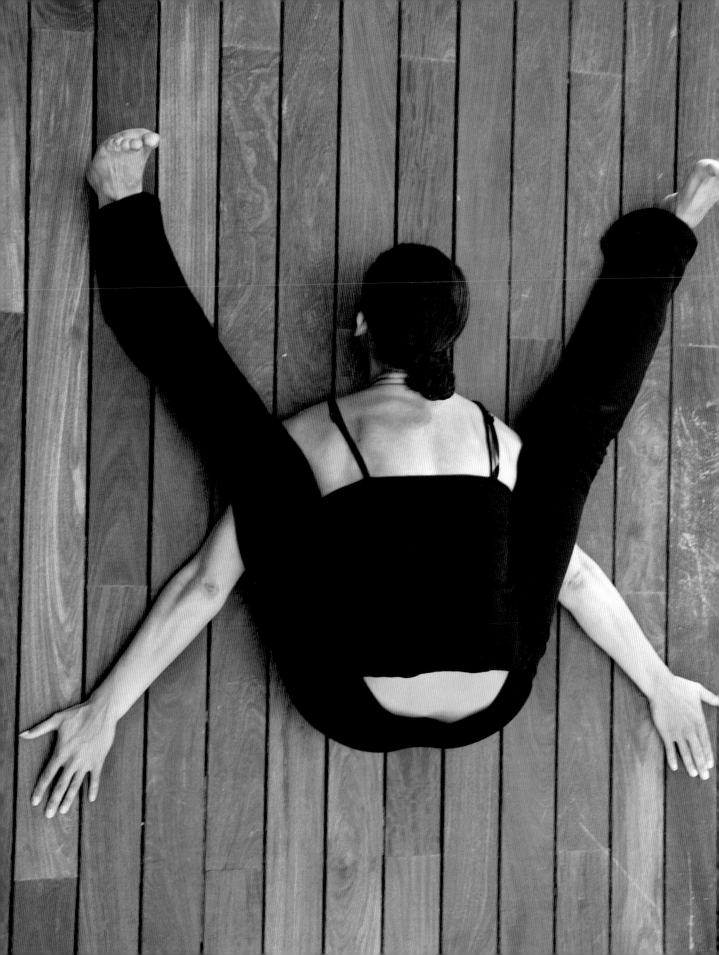

kurmasana   Tortoise Pose

This asana gives the entire back an intense stretch. The shoulders are opened and the shoulder joints limbered up. The whole spine is stretched and energized. This posture has a calming effect on the nervous system, resulting in a sense of peace.

Alignment

- Sit upright and open your legs out to each side. Bend your legs and take your arms under your knees. Inhale and lengthen through the crown of your head (see Starting posture).

- Exhale and bend forward from your hips, keeping your lower back straight. Push your tailbone back. Tense your leg muscles and push your flexed feet forward.

- Stretch your legs equally as you keep pressing further forward, at the same time pushing your arms further back.

- Continue in this way, breathing further into the posture, until your knees are pressing on your shoulders and you can rest your chin on the floor.

- Only bend as far forward as you can while keeping your lower back straight. If you round your lower back, you will lose some of the forward bend. Gradually stretch your legs while at the same time going deeper into the forward bend.

◀ *Starting posture*

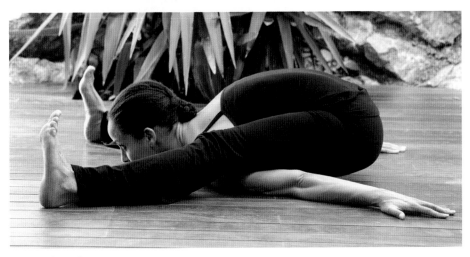

Kurmasana is a complex, demanding asana that requires not only a great deal of practice but that the muscles be well warmed-up and stretched too. So prepare for this pose with some gentle forward bends.

◀ *Side view*

◀ *View from above*

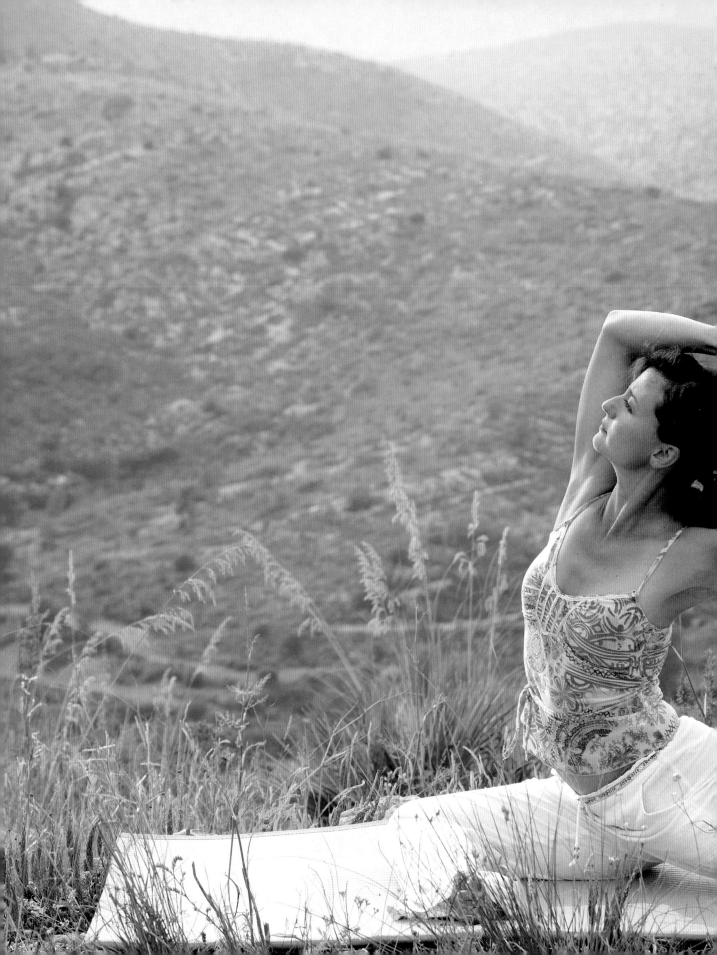

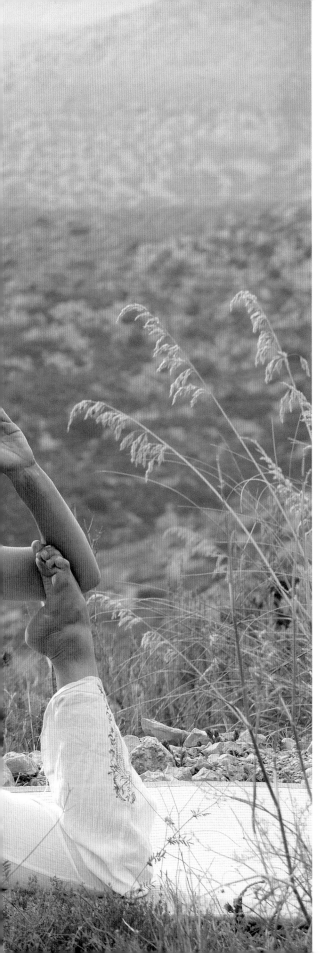

Backbends

Unlike forward bends, which dominate everyday life, backbends are not a natural movement. When practised correctly, they help with back strains, open up the chest and ensure good posture.

The movement mainly involves an even bend through the thoracic vertebrae. Because these are located in the least mobile part of the spine, the important thing is not to replace the spine's natural flexibility with excessive bending of the neck vertebrae or a hollow back, but to support it with Uddiyana bandha (see p.52).

Physiologically, the front of the body is stretched and the back is strengthened. The chest is opened up and the shoulder muscles become more flexible. Backbends energize the whole body and invigorate the central nervous system.

On an emotional level, backbends open up the heart and lift the spirits, but they sometimes require some courage. The backbend usually prevents you from looking back and demands (but also promotes) the confidence to embrace the unknown wholeheartedly.

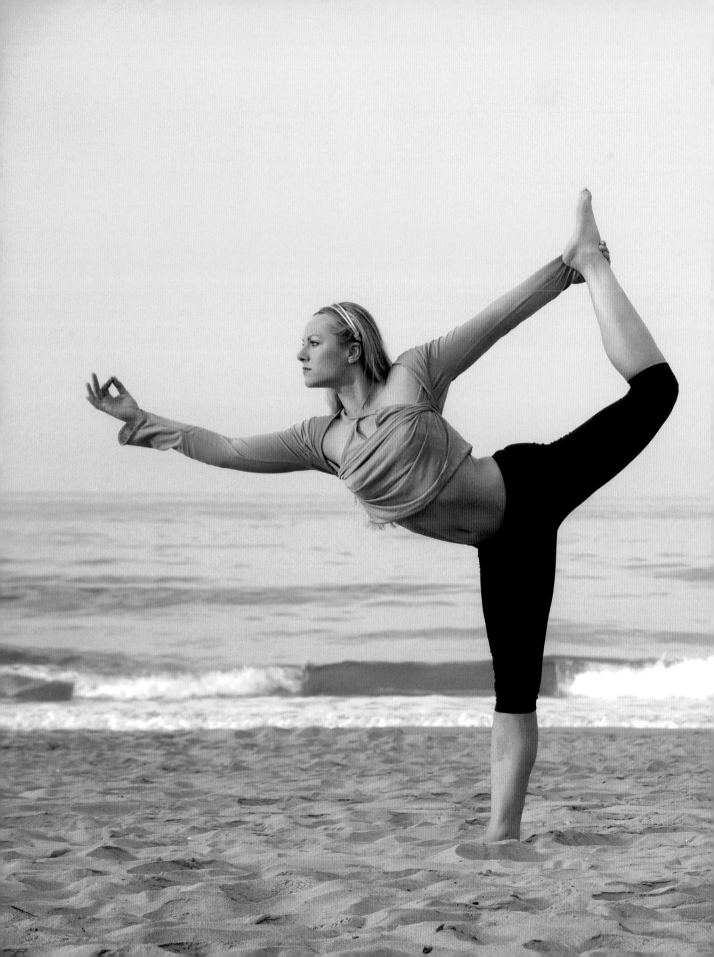

natarajasana Dancer's Pose

This graceful asana strengthens the muscles of the standing leg and stretches the front of the bent leg and the hip flexor. The chest and shoulder muscles are stretched and become more flexible. This challenging balance develops mental concentration and provides a feeling of equilibrium.

Alignment

- Find a firm position on your standing leg. Bend your other leg and raise it up behind you, grabbing your ankle with the hand of the same side.

- Inhale and lengthen up through your upper back, open up your chest, lifting the sternum, and bend gently back and down.

- As you exhale, press your raised foot into your hand and draw your bent leg up high, as if you were stretching it. Bend forward slightly, stretch your other arm forward and hold your hand in Jnana mudra (see p.39). Hold the backbend in the thoracic vertebrae and draw your tailbone gently backwards.

- Your torso should remain aligned as far forward as possible.

- Bend your neck back gently, so that your backbone is evenly curved. Bring your gaze up slightly.

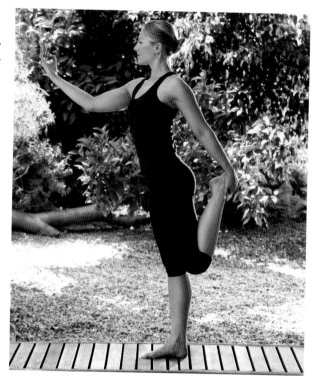

Backbends

For beginners

Begin by simply gripping your foot without raising your leg too high and focus on the backbend from your lower back.

◄ For advanced students

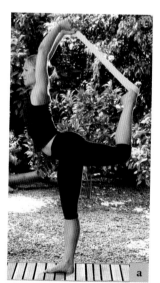
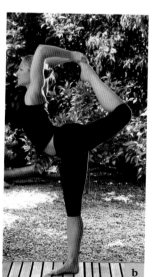

a. Place a belt around your instep and grip the belt with both hands. As you inhale, lengthen up and back from your thoracic vertebrae, at the same time using the belt to lift the leg higher. Exhale and push your tailbone back.

b. If you are flexible enough, begin by grabbing your foot with one hand and then with the other one. Your elbows should point forward and your upper arms should come alongside your ears.

virabhadrasana III Warrior Pose III

This posture strengthens the muscles in the standing leg and the trunk. The chest and shoulder muscles are stretched by the gentle backbend and therefore become more flexible. Due to the concentration required on the balance, the backbend not only energizes the body, but also provides a sense of equilibrium.

Alignment

- Find a firm position on your standing leg and keep the muscles tensed. As you inhale, stretch and raise your other leg, exhale and bend forward until your body is virtually horizontal.

- Lengthen your body as you inhale, lift your sternum and bend back from your thoracic vertebrae into an even bend.

- As you exhale, bring your arms alongside your body and push your tailbone back.

- The muscles of your extended leg should also be tensed, as if you were pushing your foot against a wall. Your toes should be pointing down and slightly inwards. Bend your neck back a little, so that your spine is evenly curved. Look upwards slightly.

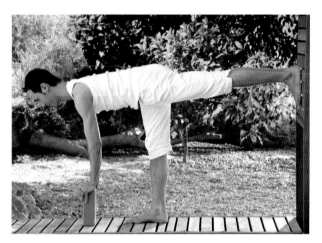

For beginners ▲

Use a block to support yourself on your hands and press the foot of your outstretched leg firmly against a wall.

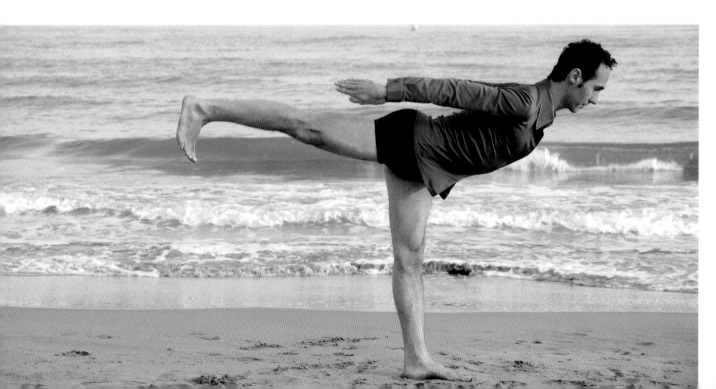

anahata asana Heart Pose

This asana opens up and intensely stretches the chest and shoulder muscles in particular, making it an ideal starting posture for deeper backbends. The whole chest cavity is opened up.

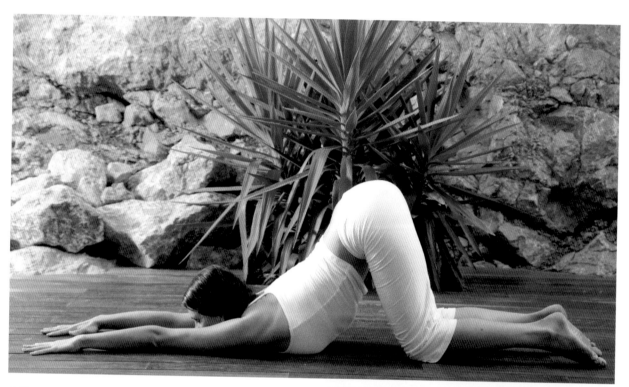

Alignment

- Get onto all fours.

- As you inhale, extend your arms forward and place your chin and chest on the floor.

- Exhale and push your tailbone up, allowing your shoulders to drop slightly lower.

- Your thighs should remain straight and your buttocks pointing up.

- Your neck should be relaxed and your gaze should be brought forward.

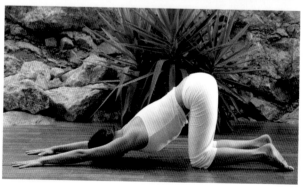

For beginners ▲

If you cannot get your chest and chin to the floor, start by simply placing your forehead on the floor.

anjaneyasana Crescent Pose

This position strengthens and stretches the fronts and backs of the legs, and the groin area. The chest and shoulder muscles are stretched, which increases their mobility. The sense of balance is challenged, combining mental concentration with a feeling of equilibrium.

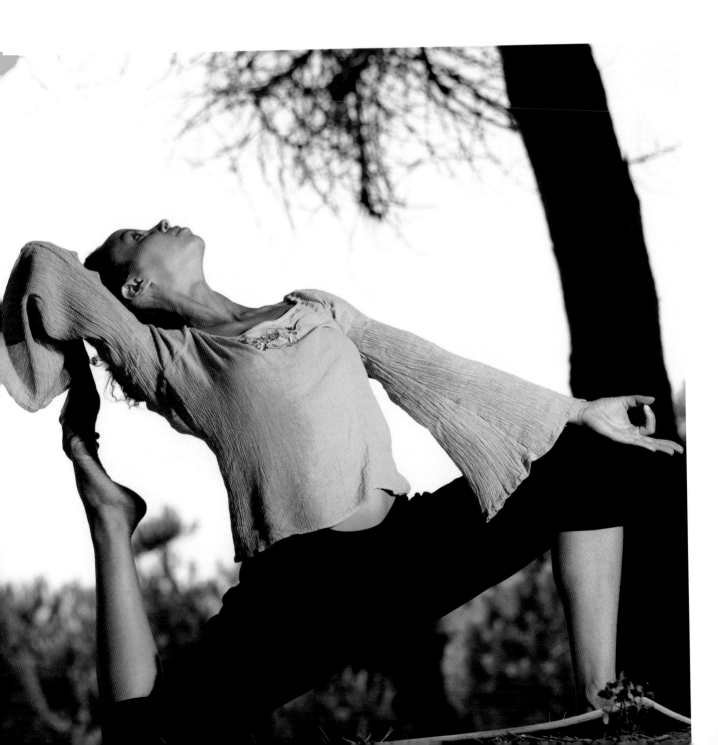

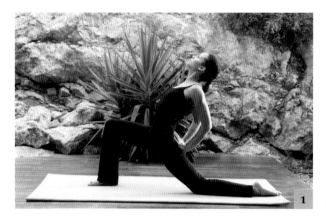
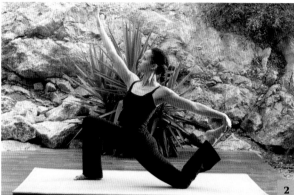

Step-by-step alignment

1. Starting in a lunge position, lower your back knee until your kneecap is touching the floor. Allow yourself to sink deeply into your hips. On an inhalation, lengthen your upper back and bend backwards. As you exhale, push your tailbone down and increase the distance between your stomach and your front leg. At the same time, place your hands on your sacrum to stop you from hollowing your back.

2. As you inhale, bend your back leg and take hold of your foot with the hand of the same side. On the exhalation, sink lower into your hips, pushing your tailbone down and pulling your navel in.

3. On the inhalation, lengthen your body again, and bend back as far as possible from your upper back. On the exhalation, pull your foot as close as possible towards your head, while sinking deeper into your hips and pushing your tailbone down further. Your hips should remain facing forward.

Variation ▼

Lay the tip of your foot in the crook of your arm and interlock your hands behind your head. Continue to keep your upper body as far forward as possible.

For beginners ▶

Remain in position 1 and practise the backbend from the upper back with arms stretched upwards.

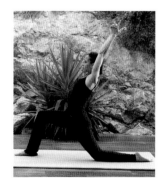

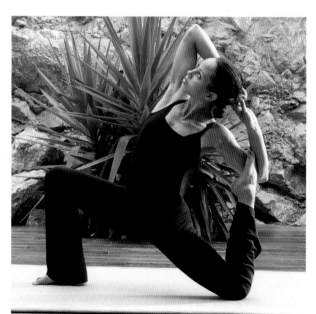

ṣhalabhāṣana Locust Pose

This asana strengthens the whole back, particularly the deep-seated muscles that keep the torso erect. It strengthens and energizes the spine, and stretches the chest and shoulder muscles. The abdominal organs are massaged, which stimulates digestion. Locust Pose can help alleviate lower back pain.

Alignment

- Lie on your front with your legs together so that your thighs, knees and ankles are all touching. Stretch your arms forward and rotate your thighs gently inwards.

- Inhale and lift your arms and legs off the floor, stretching forward through the crown of your head and back through your feet. Pull your breastbone up and bend backwards from your upper back.

- Exhale and press your pubic bone into the ground, push your tailbone towards your heels and pull your navel in towards your spine. Maintain the bend in the upper back and the long stretch.

- Your arms and legs should stay strong and your neck should bend slightly to lengthen your spine. Direct your gaze forward.

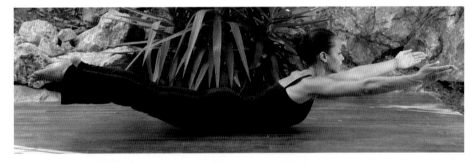

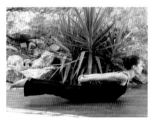

Variation ▲

Reach behind you with both arms and clasp your hands together. As you inhale, push your arms further back. This arm position strengthens the backbend and helps to open the chest cavity and shoulders.

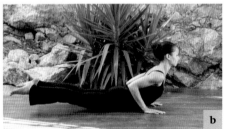

For beginners ▲

a. Alternate raising one leg and the opposite arm, supporting yourself from your shoulder with your other arm.

b. Place your hands under your shoulders and support your upper body.

Backbends

ḍhanurāṣana Bow Pose

This asana gives the whole front of the body an intense stretch and strengthens the back. It also strengthens and energizes the spine, and stretches the chest and shoulder muscles. The abdominal organs are massaged, stimulating digestion. Lower back pain can be alleviated by this asana.

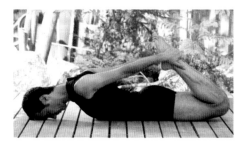

Starting posture

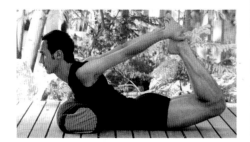

For beginners ▲

Place a cushion under your chest if you are unable to raise your upper body from the floor.

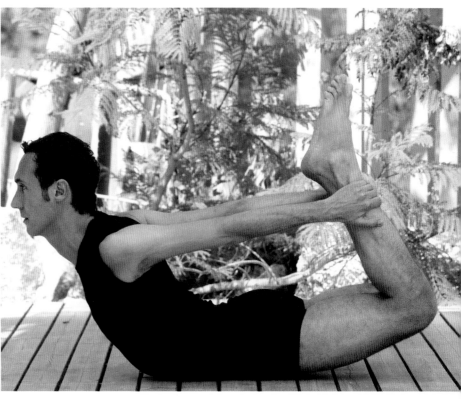

Alignment

- Lie flat on your stomach. Put your legs together so that your thighs, knees and ankles are all touching. If you are unable to do this, open your knees, but no further than hip-width apart. Bend your legs, and reaching back with your hands, take hold of your ankles (see Starting posture).

- As you inhale, lift your breastbone up and bend your upper back towards your feet, raising your arms and legs from the floor at the same time. Keep pressing your feet into your hands, as if trying to stretch your legs.

- As you exhale, push your pubic bone into the ground, pull your navel in and push your tailbone back. Maintain the backbend in the upper back.

- Bend your neck back gently, so that your spine forms an even bow. Direct your gaze forward.

उष्ट्रासन ushtrasana Camel Pose

This asana gives the whole front of the body an intense stretch and strengthens the back. It energizes the spine, and stretches the chest and shoulder muscles. Lung volume is increased and body posture improved.

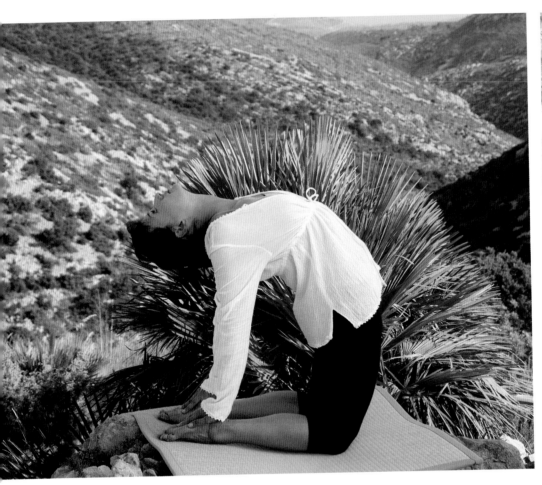

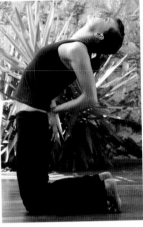

For beginners ▲

Place your hands on your sacrum and bend back to the point where you can keep your thighs upright – pressed against an imaginary wall.

Only allow your head to fall back onto your shoulder muscles if you do not suffer from neck problems.

Alignment

- Assume a kneeling position. Tense your thigh muscles, turn your thighs inward slightly and push them forward as if pressing them against a wall. Stay upright and maintain this tension, keeping the pelvis straight.

- As you inhale, pull yourself up through the crown of your head, lift your breastbone and bend backwards from your thoracic vertebrae.

- On exhaling, reach both arms back and grasp your ankles – or lay your hands flat on the soles of your feet. Push your tailbone down, pull your pubic bone up and relax your head back onto your neck.

- Inhale and come out of the position.

꫱ꫀꩅꪊ ꪚꪖꪀꪗꪜꪖꪤꪖꪀꪖ   **Bridge Pose**

This asana gives the whole front of the body an intense stretch and strengthens the back. The chest and shoulder muscles are also stretched. The upper thighs are strengthened too and the spine is energized.

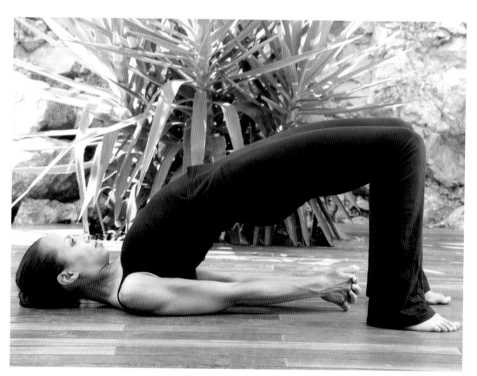

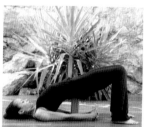

For beginners ▲

Place a block immediately under your sacrum if you cannot hold your body up.

Alignment

- Lie with your back flat on the floor. Open your knees no further than hip-width apart and place the heels of your feet close to your buttocks.

- As you inhale, raise your pelvis and push it upwards to stretch the groin area. Push your breastbone towards your chin. Fold your hands under your body, and press your upper arms and feet firmly down on the floor.

- On an exhalation, push your tailbone towards your knees. Maintain the bend in the upper back.

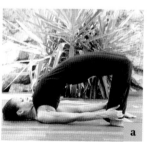

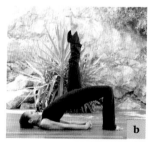

For advanced students ▲

a. Take hold of your ankles with your hands to strengthen the bend.

b. Stretch one leg straight up in the air to challenge your sense of balance and strengthen the core of your body and your lower leg.

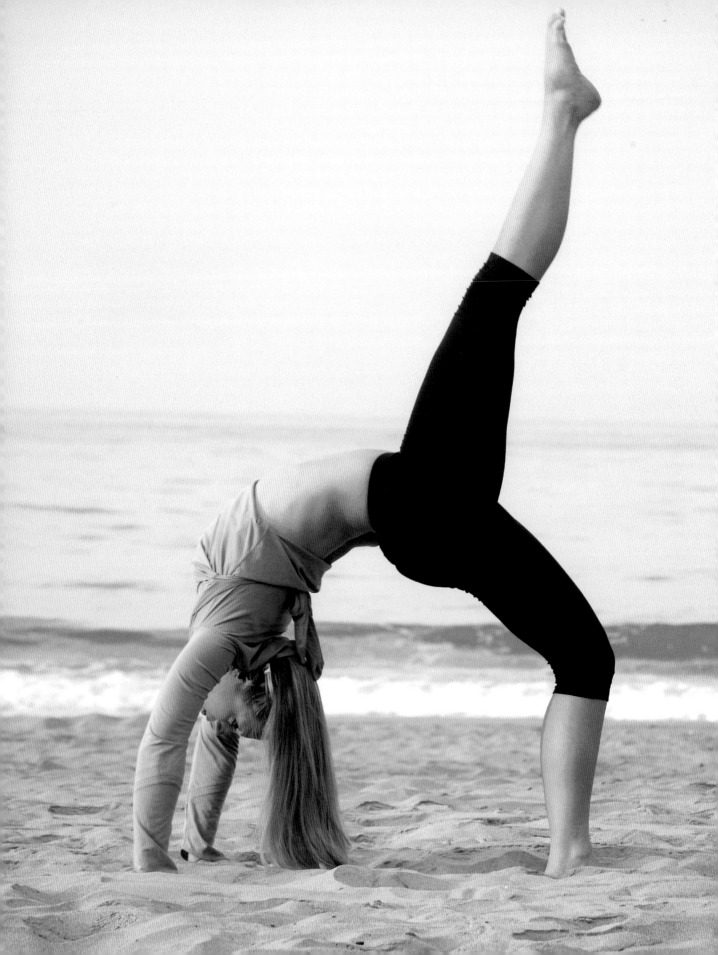

उर्ध्व धनुरासन   Wheel Pose

This asana gives the whole front of the body an intense stretch and strengthens the back. It energizes the spine, and stretches the chest and shoulder muscles. At the same time, lung volume is increased and body posture improved.

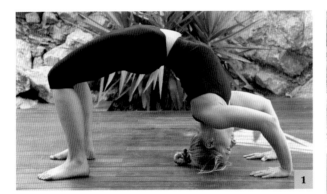

Step-by-step alignment

1. Lie with your back flat on the floor. Open your knees no further than hip-width apart and place the heels of your feet close to your buttocks. The outer edges of your feet should be parallel. Place your hands alongside your head, so that your fingertips are under the top of your shoulders. Keep your elbows as close together as possible.

   - As you inhale, push down through your hands and feet and lift your whole body up from the floor, pushing your pelvis up.

   - As you exhale, lower the crown of your head to the ground, but keep your pelvis up. Push your tailbone further back and your elbows together.

2. Increase the pressure through your hands and feet and stretch through your thoracic vertebrae.

   - On an inhalation, lift your pelvis and breastbone at the same time as stretching your arms. Your head will automatically come up from the ground. Make sure your neck remains relaxed, your arms stay close to your body and your shoulder blades are drawn inwards.

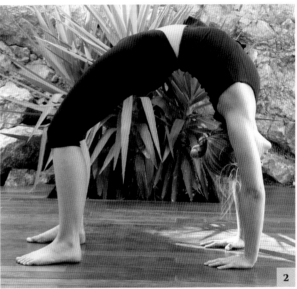

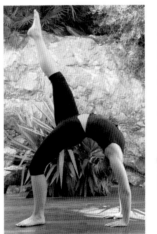

◄ For advanced students

Raise alternate legs and continue to keep your weight evenly distributed between your hands and the foot that remains on the floor.

Urdhva Dhanurasana is an intense backbend. Only practise it once you have warmed up with some easier backbends and prepared your body sufficiently.

   - Push your tailbone down towards your knees and press your thighs together. Distribute your weight evenly between your hands and feet.

ꚛupta Virāꚛana Supine Hero Pose

This asana gives the entire front of the body, in particular the fronts of the thighs, an intense stretch. It makes the knee joints supple and alleviates the feeling of heavy legs. With a certain amount of practice, the position becomes relaxing, as well as providing the energizing effect of a backward bend.

Alignment

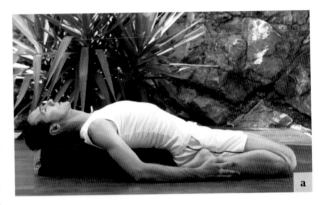

- Sit upright in Virasana (see p.204). As you inhale, straighten your spine, and on an exhalation, lie back onto your lower arms, then onto your back. Support yourself by positioning your hands next to your thighs.

- Lift your breastbone, maintaining the length in your spine. Rest your arms comfortably alongside your body.

- Push your tailbone back and squeeze your thighs together to prevent your knees from spreading. Press the tops of your feet into the floor.

- Continue breathing normally and relax into the position. Turn your knees inwards.

- Come out of the position on an exhalation.

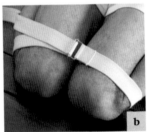

For beginners

a. Place a large cushion behind your buttocks if you are not able to recline onto your back.

b. Tie a belt around your legs if you cannot keep your thighs and knees together.

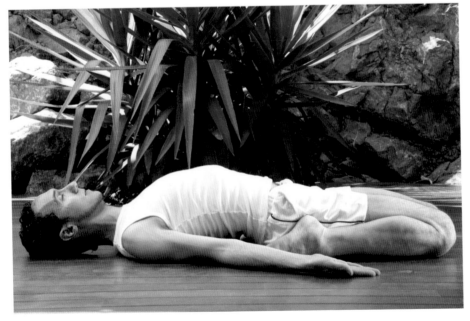

> Only practise Supta Virasana when you can sit comfortably on the floor in Virasana (see p.204) without using a block.

ᜋᜆᜌᜐᜈ Fish Pose

This asana stretches the front of the body and opens the shoulders and chest. The upper back and neck muscles are strengthened. At the same time, circulation to the pelvis is increased and the knees become more supple.

Alignment

- Lie flat on the floor and fold your legs in Padmasana (see p.206). Place your thumbs under your buttocks.

- Lengthen your spine as you breathe in and pull the breastbone up, supporting yourself on your forearms as you do so.

- As you exhale, lower the crown of your head to the floor and push your tailbone towards your legs; this prevents you from hollowing your back. Hold the pose, keeping the length and backbend in the thoracic vertebrae.

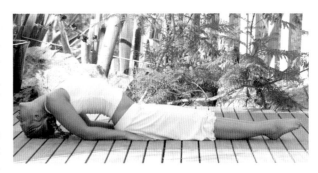

For beginners ▲

If you are not yet able to sit in Padmasana, keep your legs stretched out straight on the floor with your toes pointed forward.

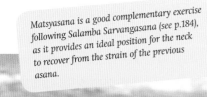

Matsyasana is a good complementary exercise following Salamba Sarvangasana (see p.184), as it provides an ideal position for the neck to recover from the strain of the previous asana.

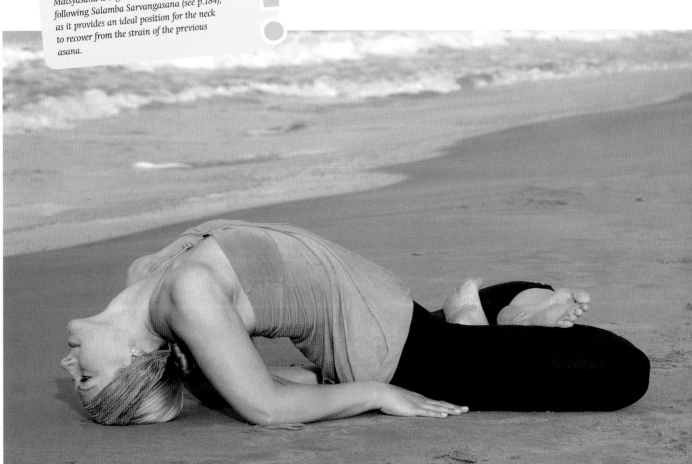

eka pada rajakapotasana One-Legged King Pigeon Pose

The whole spine is energized in this asana. As you bend back, it also creates an intense stretch to the fronts of the legs, the groin and the buttocks. The chest and shoulder muscles are stretched. This position brings a sense of vitality and energy to the body.

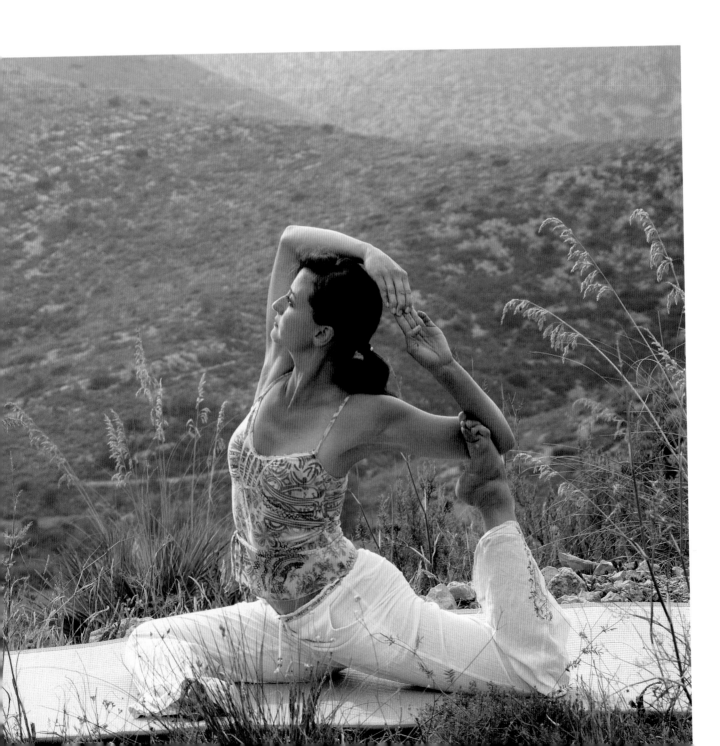

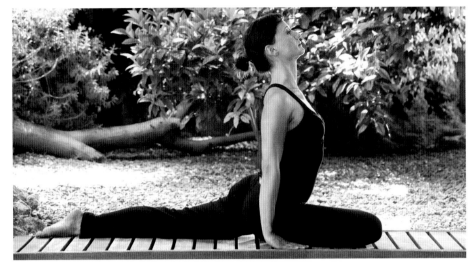

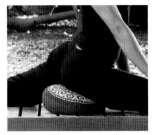

For beginners ▲

Position a cushion below the hip of your front leg if you find yourself tipping to one side. This keeps your hips parallel.

Starting posture

Alignment

- From a sitting position, bend one knee in front of you and stretch the other leg straight behind you. Your front thigh, shin and the top of your foot should lie centrally and your rear foot should be pointed straight back. Your hips should be parallel and facing forward (see Starting posture). Your feet should be pressed into the ground.

- On an inhalation, pull yourself up through the crown of your head from your thoracic vertebrae and bend gently backwards. At the same time, bend your back leg, draw the arm on the same side back, and place your foot in the crook of your arm.

- As you exhale, take your other arm back past your head and take hold of your other hand with this hand. Push your tailbone down and sink lower into your hips. Try to keep your upper body facing forward. The foot of your front leg should press into the ground to keep you stable.

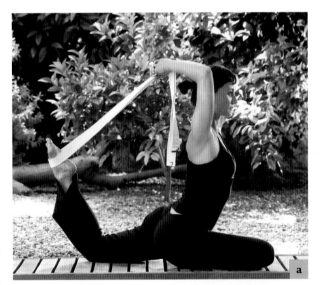

For advanced students ▶

a. Put a belt around your foot and take hold of it with both hands. As you inhale, pull yourself up and back from your thoracic vertebrae, using the belt to pull your rear leg higher. As you exhale, push your tailbone down.

b. If you are flexible enough, grab your back foot with both hands. Your elbows should remain forward and your upper arms should be directly next to the ears.

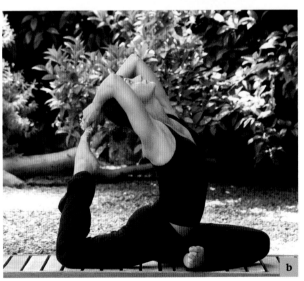

bhekasana Frog Pose

This asana stretches the entire front of the body, particularly the fronts of the thighs, groin and shoulders. Pressing down into the floor massages the abdominal organs. This posture strengthens the back and helps make the knee and foot joints supple.

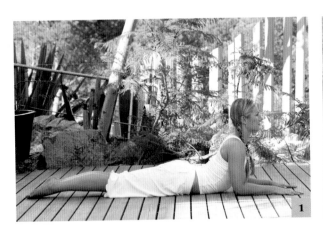

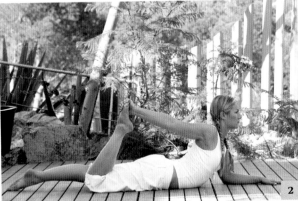

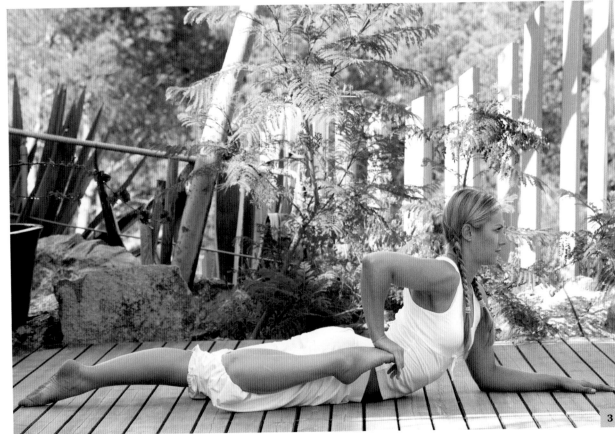

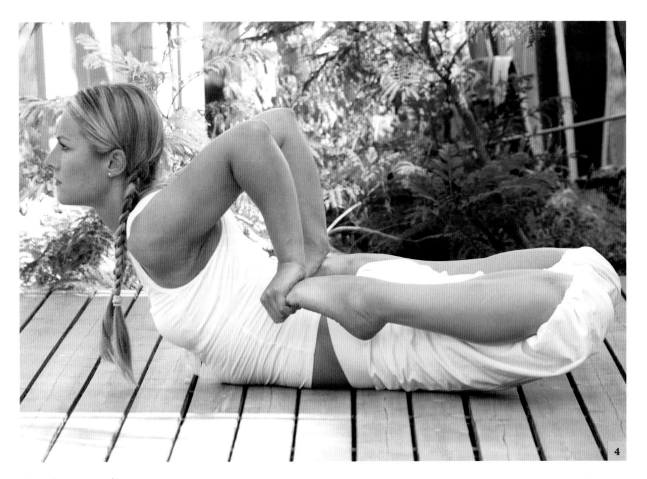

4

Step-by-step alignment

1. Lie on your front and stretch your legs straight behind you, the soles of your feet facing upwards. As you inhale, lengthen your spine, raise your upper body and rest on your lower arms. Your elbows should be directly below your shoulders. This position is also called the 'Sphinx'. As you exhale, push your pubic bone into the floor, draw your navel in and push your tailbone back.

2. As you inhale, bend one leg. Pull yourself up and back from your upper spine, at the same time drawing back the arm on the same side and taking hold of your foot.

3. Exhale and rotate your shoulder inwards, so that your elbow is facing up and back. At the same time, turn your hand towards the front and place the palm of your hand on the top of your foot. Press your foot gently towards the ground.

4. Repeat steps 2 and 3 with the other leg. As you do so, squeeze your thighs together so that your knees do not drift apart. Keep the length in your spine.

Bhekasana is a complex position that requires your body to be sufficiently warmed up and stretched. Prepare yourself with easy, but similar, postures, e.g. Ushtrasana (see p.132) or Supta Virasana (see p.136). Or start by practising with alternate legs, before bending them both at the same time.

॑hanumanasana Monkey Pose

Besides being a strong backbend, this asana gives the backs and fronts of the legs an intense stretch. The hips are opened and blood circulation around the hips is improved. Monkey Pose can help to alleviate sciatic problems and the feeling of heavy legs. The posture stretches the front of the body and strengthens the back.

Alignment

- From a kneeling position, first stretch one leg straight in front of you and then the other straight behind.

- Keep your upper body central over your hips and carefully push your front leg further forward and your back leg further back, until your crotch is touching the floor.

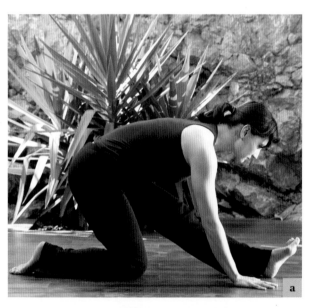

- Use your hands to support you. Both legs should remain tense, with your front foot pulled towards you and your back foot resting on your toes until your crotch is touching the floor.

- Once both legs are straight, inhale and stretch up through your spine as you raise your arms above your head. As you exhale, push your tailbone down and sink lower into your hips. Maintain the stretch of the spine.

◀ For beginners

a. Start by practising the half splits (Ardha Hanumanasana), by resting one leg in a kneeling position and working on the stretch of the thigh muscles at the back of the front leg.

b. If you cannot lower your crotch to the floor, relieve the pressure on your legs by resting your weight on a block, bending forward and supporting yourself on your hands. You can also position blocks under your hands and sit up straight.

c. Once you are able to go lower, but not quite down to the ground, sit on a cushion.

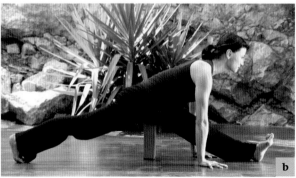

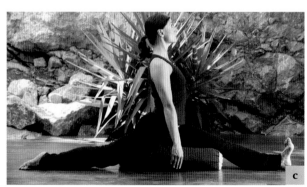

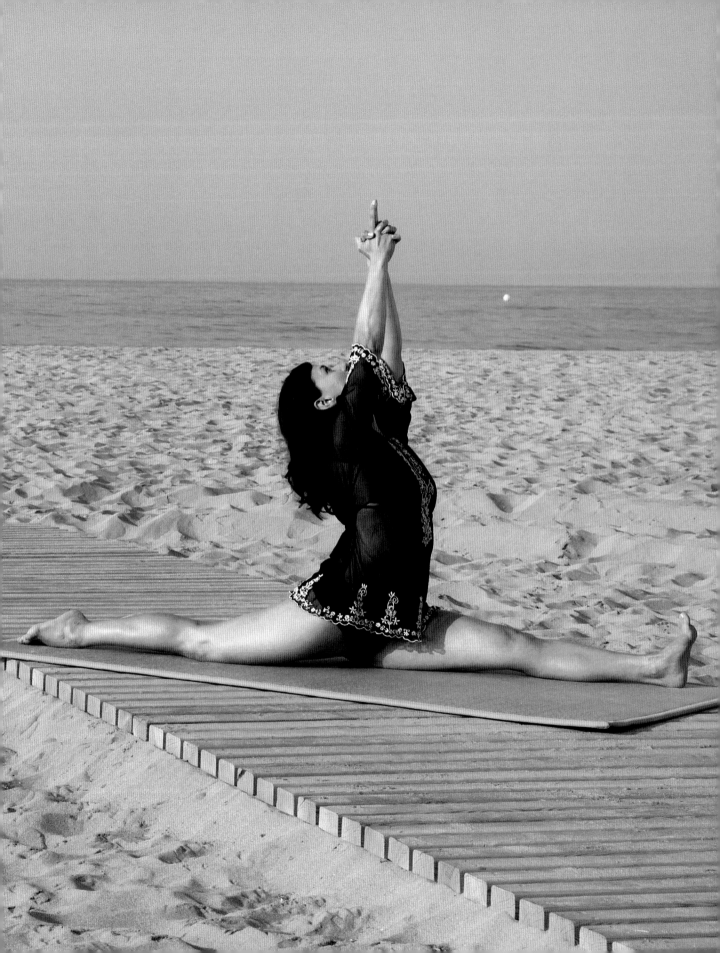

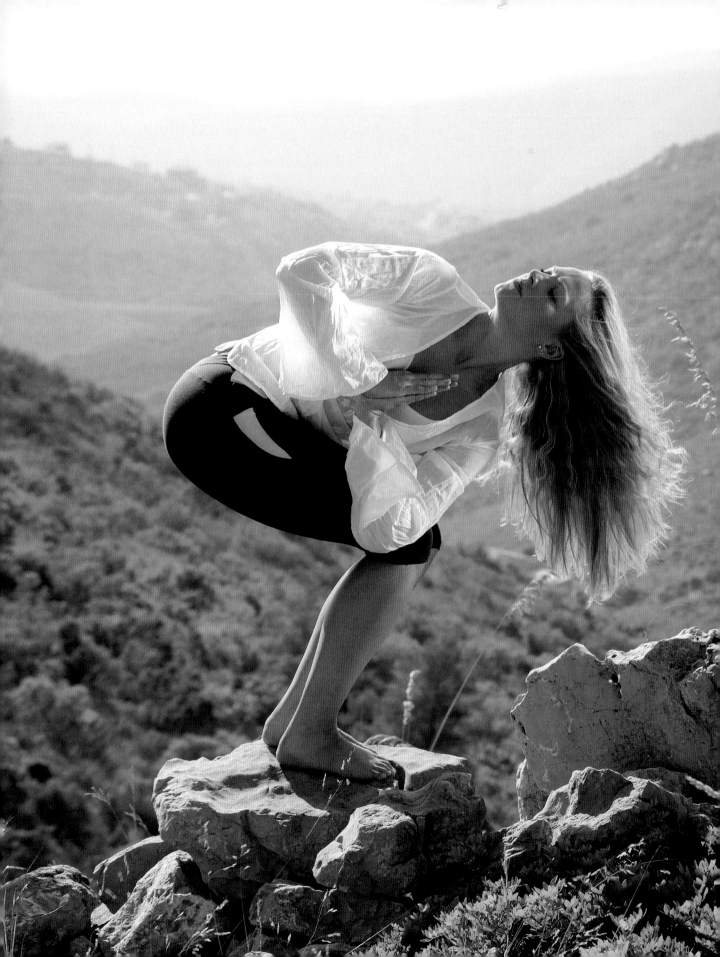

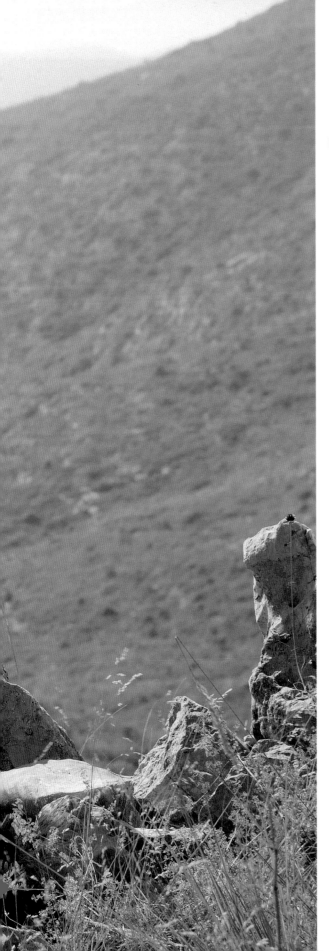

Twists

Twists are rotations around the centre axis of the body and the spine. The twisting motion around the spine, which should be held in a lengthened position, comes mainly from the thoracic vertebrae. The pelvis does not rotate, but remains parallel. Twists should always be practised on both sides – first to the right, then to the left.

The physiological benefit of twists is that they massage and stimulate the digestive organs, helping to regulate digestion. Gentle twists can also release tensions after intense backward or forward bends and neutralize the spine.

On an emotional level, twists help to cultivate a feeling of inner peace, even in awkward situations. They give you the means to be able to find space even in a confined area, and allow you to relax and deal with a situation calmly.

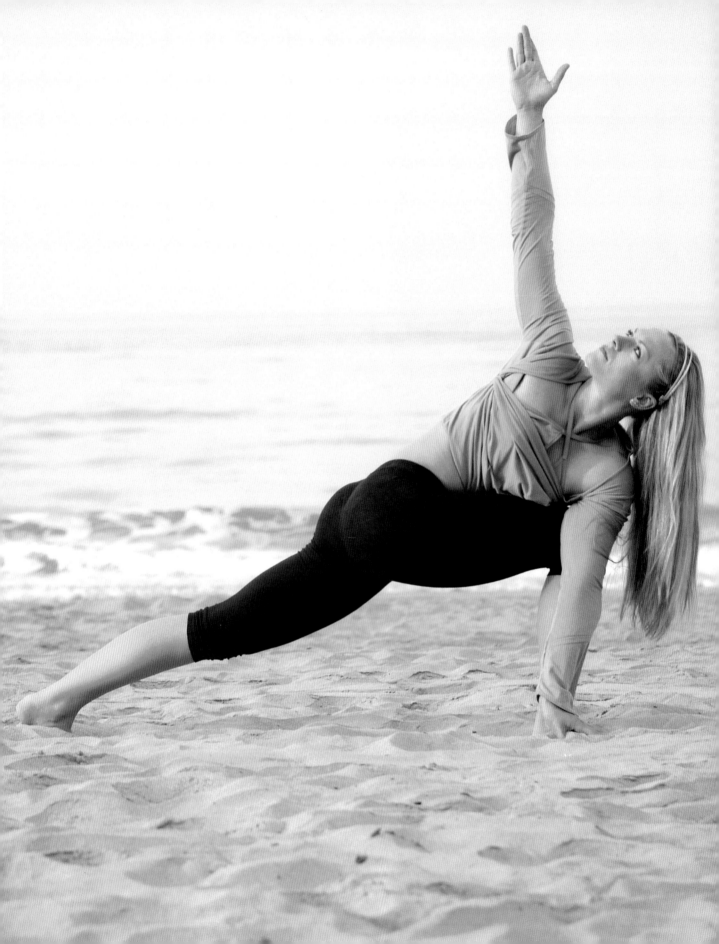

parivritta parsvakonasana   Revolved Side Angle Pose

This asana is particularly beneficial for strengthening and stretching the thigh muscles. Blood circulation to the digestive organs is improved, as the organs are massaged and stimulated by the twisting motion and the pressure of the front leg. This improves digestion and literally 'wrings' waste materials out of the body. The twist also strengthens and energizes the spine.

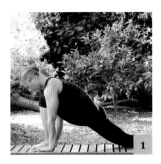 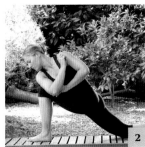 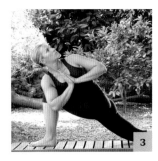 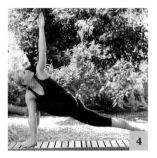

Step-by-step alignment

1. Step back as far as you can and allow your back knee to sink to the ground.

2. As you inhale, lengthen your spine through the crown of your head, and as you exhale, turn yourself in the direction of your front knee. Place your upper arm on the outside of the knee.

3. On your next inhalation, lengthen your spine again and press gently with your upper arm against the outside of your knee, placing the palms of your hands together.

4. As you exhale, place your lower hand flat on the floor beside the outer edge of your front foot, raise your back knee from the ground and stretch the leg behind you. Open up your thoracic spine to the side and take your upper arm straight up. Look up at your hand.

For beginners   ▶

a. Leave your knee on the ground and place your front hand flat on the inner edge of your front foot.

b. Place your front hand on a block next to the outer edge of your front foot and rest your other hand on your hip.

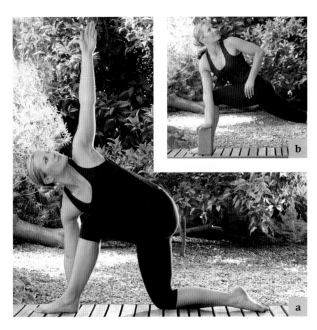

parivritta trikonasana
Revolved Triangle Pose

This asana is particularly beneficial for strengthening the thigh and calf muscles. It also strengthens the hip muscles. Blood circulation to the lower abdomen and the lower part of the spine is improved, thereby stimulating the digestive organs and regulating digestion. The twisting motion energizes the spine.

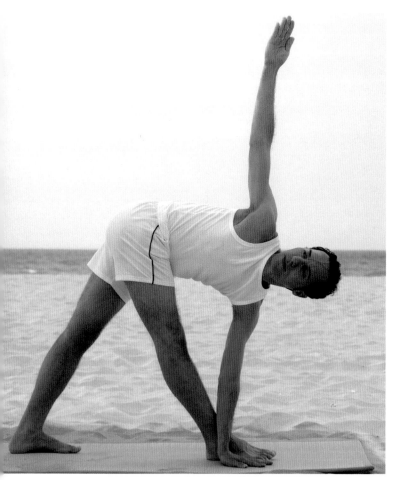

Alignment

- Step forward by about 1 metre (3 feet) and keep both feet and your hips facing forwards. Tense the muscles in your legs.

- Keeping your back straight, bend your upper body forward by an angle of about 90 degrees.

- As you inhale, lengthen your spine and push your tailbone back.

- As you exhale, take the hand on the opposite side to the front leg down beside the outer edge of your front foot and twist to the side, bringing your other arm up above you, and directing your gaze at your outstretched arm. Keep your spine lengthened.

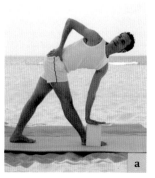
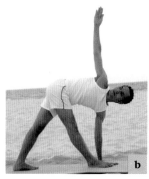

For beginners ▲

a. If you cannot reach the ground with your supporting hand, put a block beside the outer edge of your foot and place your hand on it. With your other hand, take hold of the hip of your front leg and gently push back.

b. Place your hand beside the inner edge of your front foot and stretch your other arm up above you.

This asana places particular strain on the hamstrings, so it is essential that you ensure that the knee of your front leg is not stretched too far.

parivritta ardha chandrasana
Revolved Half Moon Pose

This asana is particularly beneficial for strengthening the thigh, hip and buttock muscles. Blood circulation to the lower abdomen and the lower part of the spine is stimulated, thereby stimulating the digestive organs and regulating digestion. The twisting motion also energizes the spine. This asana can help to improve the sense of balance.

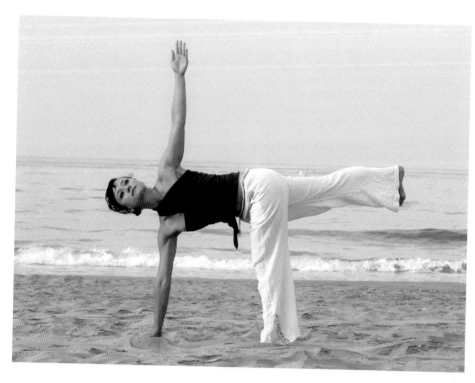

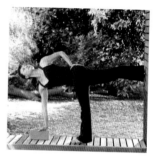

For beginners ▲

Place your supporting hand on a block and press your back leg firmly against a wall. Rest your upper hand on your hip and push gently backwards.

Alignment

- Ground your standing leg and distribute your weight over the whole foot. This foot should be pointing straight ahead.

- As you inhale, stretch forward with your opposite hand by about 30 cm (10 inches), making the shape of a tent. Raise your other leg and stretch it straight out behind you. Your toes should point to the floor and your hips remain parallel. Stretch forward through the crown of your head and back through your raised foot. Your tailbone should pull in the direction of your back heel.

- As you exhale, turn your upper body to the side and bring your other arm straight up above you. Pull gently downwards with your supporting arm; this arm should provide stability, but should bear hardly any weight.

- Keep your shoulders relaxed and open, your arms forming a vertical line.

- Direct your gaze upwards.

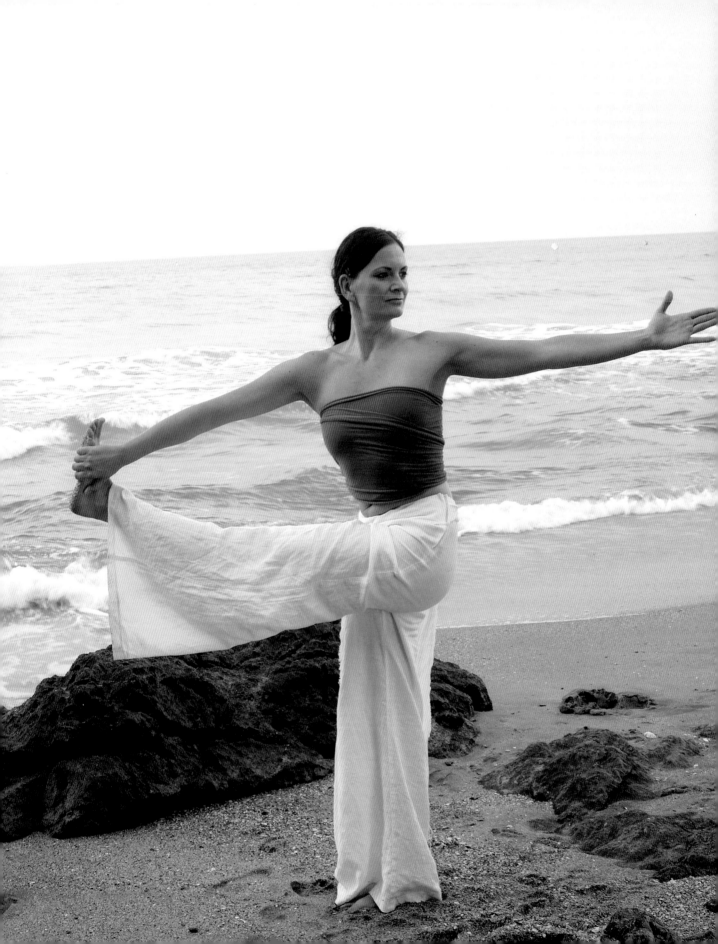

parivritta hasta padangusthasana
Revolved Hand to Toe Pose

This position is extremely beneficial for strengthening all of the leg and buttock muscles. It also gives a particularly deep stretch to the muscle at the back of the thigh of the raised leg. The twisting motion stimulates the digestive organs and energizes the spine. This asana also enhances the sense of balance.

Alignment

- Ground your standing leg and distribute your weight over your whole foot.

- Bend your other leg and take hold of the outer edge of the foot with your opposite arm. Keep your hips parallel. Stretch your other arm up (see Starting posture).

- As you inhale, stretch your bent leg out to the front, and lengthen your spine by stretching through the crown of your head and pushing your tailbone down.

- As you exhale, turn towards the leg stretched out in front of you and extend your upper arm back. Maintain your erect posture and keep your spine lengthened.

- Your gaze should follow your arm as it stretches backwards.

For beginners ▼

a. Leave your raised leg bent and steady it at the knee with your opposite hand. Take your other arm back and follow it with your eyes. Look to the front if your sense of balance does not allow you to do this yet.

b. Use a belt to help you to stretch your bent leg out.

Starting posture

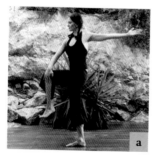

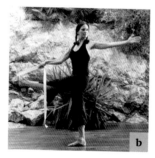

parivritta prasarita padottanasana
Revolved Wide Leg Stretch

This asana strengthens all of the muscles at the front of the legs and the buttocks. It also gives a deep stretch to the muscles at the back of the thighs and calves. The intense twisting motion stimulates the digestive organs and improves digestion. This is also a position from which you can twist a long way on both sides without having to change your leg position.

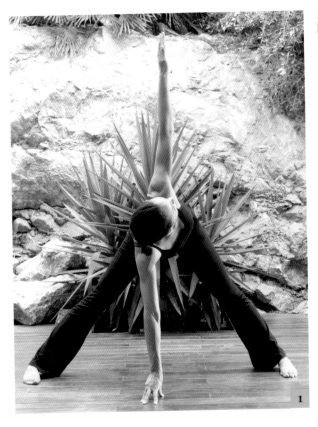

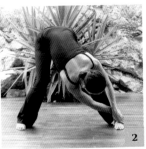
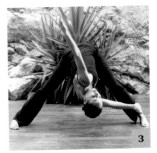

Step-by-step alignment

1. Stand with your legs wide apart, keeping both feet pointing forward. As you exhale, keep your back straight and bend forward from your hips until your upper body is horizontal. As you inhale, place one hand in front of you in the centre of the ground and lengthen your spine. As you exhale, twist your body to the side, and at the same time raise your other arm up to the ceiling.

2. As you inhale, grasp the opposite ankle with your lower hand. Bring your other arm down, and as you exhale, draw yourself gently into the leg.

3. On an inhalation, stretch your spine again. Leave your lower hand on the ankle, and as you exhale, turn to the side again and raise your other arm up to the ceiling.

4. Keep your lower hand on your ankle. As you inhale, reach down and place your raised arm between the other arm and your leg. Grasp your opposite ankle and, as you exhale, twist to the other side.

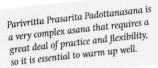

Parivritta Prasarita Padottanasana is a very complex asana that requires a great deal of practice and flexibility, so it is essential to warm up well.

Twists

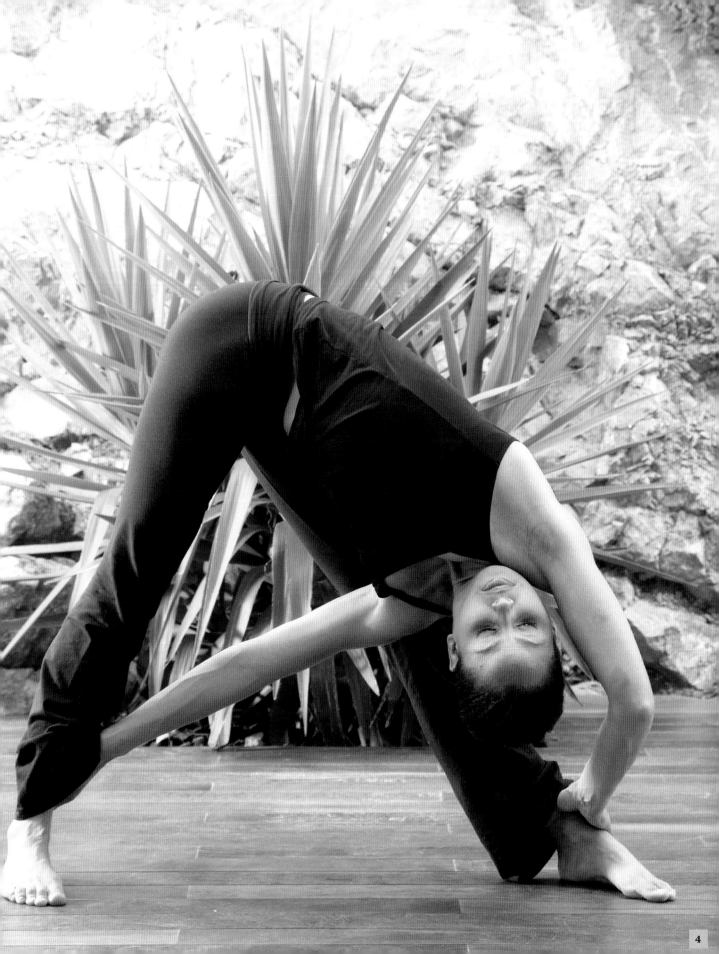

parivritta utkatasana
Revolved Fierce Pose

This asana – also called Parsva Utkatasana (Sideways Fierce Pose) – strengthens the entire lower body. The leg muscles and ankles are strengthened and the calves stretched. The twisting motion stimulates the digestive organs.

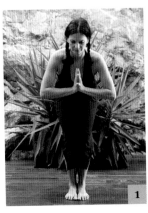 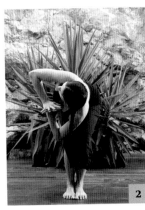

Step-by-step alignment

1. Assume the Utkatasana pose (see p.81). As you inhale, take your hands in front of your chest, lengthening your spine as you pull up through the crown of your head and push your tailbone down.

2. Exhaling, bring one elbow to the outer side of the opposite knee and twist to the side. Your knees and hips should remain parallel and at the same height.

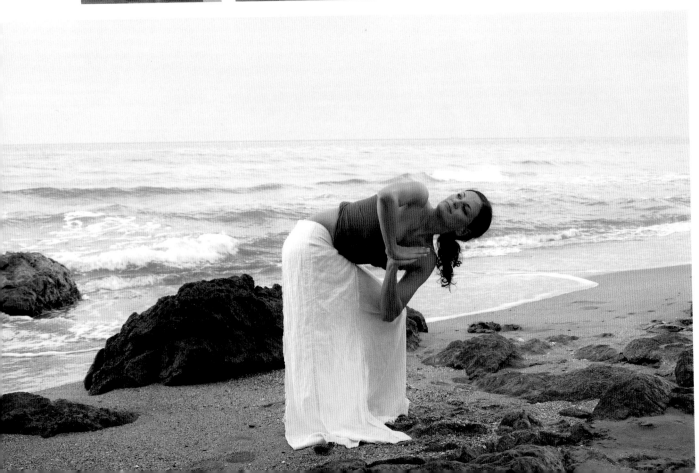

parivritta janu shirshasana
Revolved Head to Knee Pose

This asana strengthens the leg muscles and gives both the leg muscles and the sides of the body an intense stretch. It also stimulates the blood circulation to the digestive organs and improves digestion.

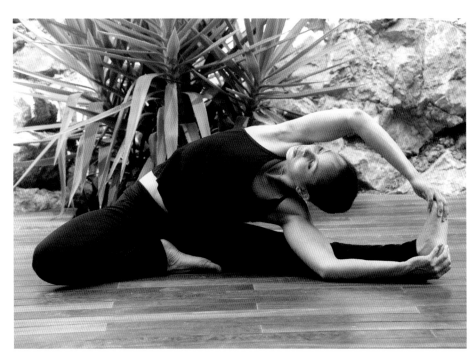
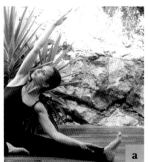
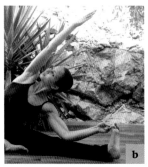

Alignment

- Start by sitting on the floor with your legs stretched out to each side. Bend one leg and bring the heel of your foot as close as possible to your pubic bone. The muscles of your outstretched leg should be as tensed as they would be standing on the floor.

- As you inhale, bend over your outstretched leg, pulling forwards through the crown of your head and pushing your tailbone back. Lay your lower forearm alongside the outstretched leg and grasp your heel with your hand.

- As you exhale, twist to the side and take hold of the toes of the outstretched leg with your other hand. Look upwards.

For beginners

a. If you are unable to grasp the foot of your outstretched leg, lay your lower arm along your shin. Extend your other arm into the air following the line of the stretched side of your body.

b. Use your lower hand to take hold of the big toe of your outstretched leg and rest your elbow between your knee and shin. Extend your other arm into the air following the line of the stretched side of your body.

Twists

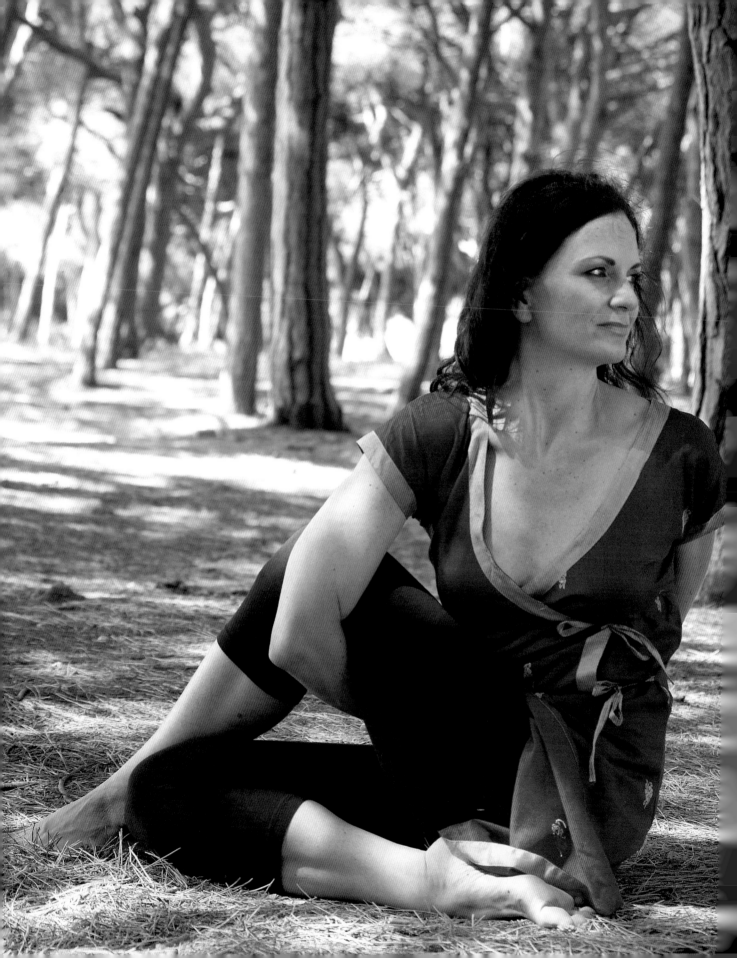

ardha matsyendrasana Half Spinal Twist

This asana improves the flexibility of the whole body. The leg muscles as well as the buttock and hip muscles are stretched, and the twist energizes the spine. It also stimulates blood circulation to the digestive organs and regulates digestion. It addition, this posture relaxes the shoulders and shoulder joints, increasing their suppleness.

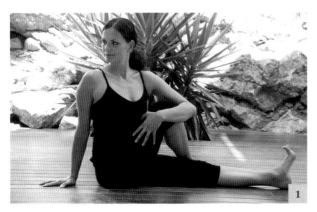

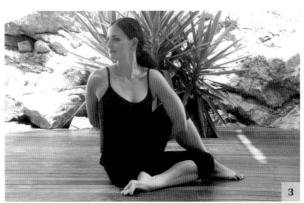

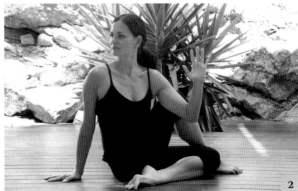

Step-by-step alignment

1. Sit upright with your legs outstretched, bend one leg and cross it over the other, placing the foot flat on the floor. Keep the muscles of your outstretched leg taut. As you inhale, lengthen your spine, and as you exhale, turn to the side and support your back by placing the hand that is further back flat on the floor. Use the forearm of your front arm to apply gentle pressure to the outer edge of your front knee.

2. Maintain the breathing pattern. Now bend your other leg and take your foot to the other side, resting the top of your foot against your buttock. Bring your front upper arm to the outside of your upright knee.

3. Rotate the shoulder of your front arm, bend this arm and reach back between your legs. Turn the shoulder of your back arm out, bend it and take it behind your back. Grasp the wrist of your back arm with the hand of your front arm. As you inhale, continue to lengthen your spine, and as you exhale, relax deeper into the twist.

Each stage of the step-by-step alignment is good for practising. If one of your hips rises from the floor, sit on a block to keep your hips parallel. However, you must then support yourself by placing your back hand on the floor.

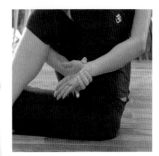

View from behind

||bharadvajasana|| Bharadvaja's Twist

There are different variations of this asana: in the Lotus position, Half Lotus, Half Lotus and Half Hero, or with bent legs next to each other. The more complex the sitting position, the greater the effect on the suppleness and flexibility of the knee and shoulder joints. The intense twist energizes and strengthens the spine in all of the variations.

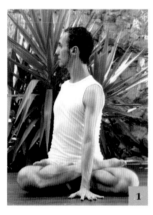

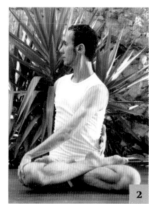

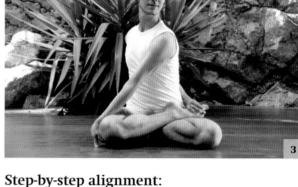

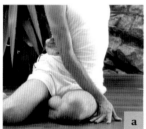

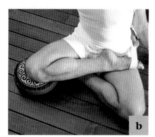

For beginners ▲

a. Bharadvajasana with legs next to each other: bend both legs to one side beneath you and then practise the twist.

b. Bharadvajasana in Half Lotus: if you are at this stage, practise the pose in Half Lotus. If necessary, place a cushion under the knee of your uppermost leg and use a belt around your foot.

Step-by-step alignment: Bharadvajasana in the Lotus position

1. Begin by sitting in the Lotus position (see p.206). As you inhale, lengthen your spine, pulling up through the crown of your head, and as you exhale, rotate through your spine and twist to one side. Place one hand in front of you and the other behind you to help you maintain the position.

2. Inhaling, continue to lengthen your spine, and as you exhale, go deeper into the twist. Place your front hand on your knee and take your other hand round behind your back, then bring it back around to the front.

3. Maintain the breathing pattern, and as you exhale, take hold of your upper foot with your back hand. Push your front hand under the knee of the same leg. Look in the opposite direction of the twist so that your spine twists round twice like a corkscrew.

Bharadvajasana in Half Lotus (see p.206) and Half Hero (see p.204) ▶

Twists

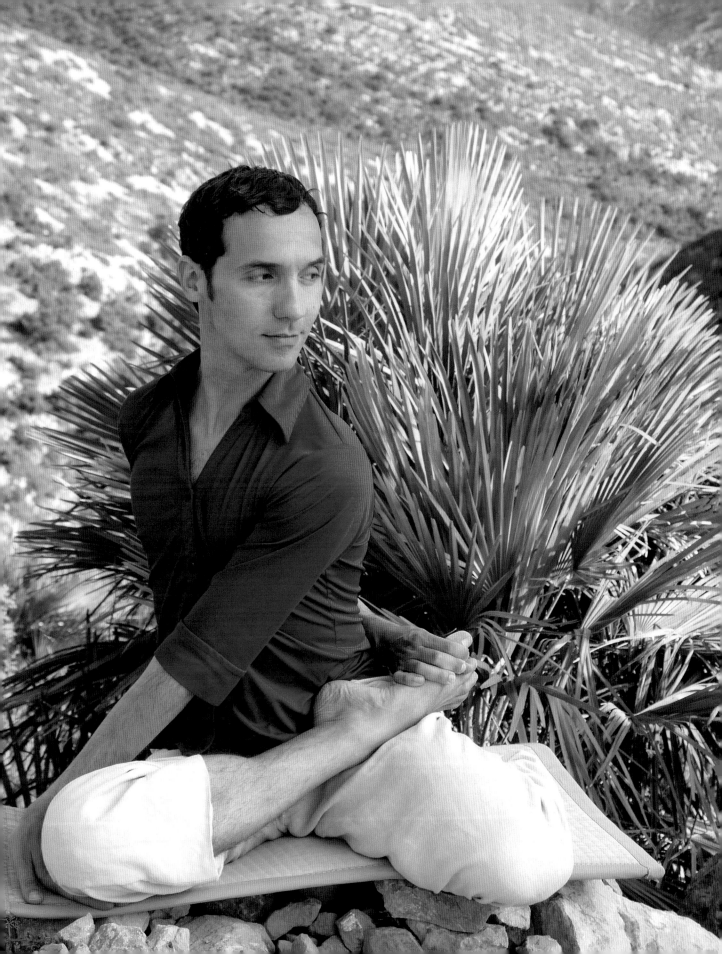

मारिच्यासन ८ Marichi's Pose C

This asana improves the flexibility of the whole body. The leg muscles and the muscles of the buttock and hip region are stretched. The twist has an energizing effect on the spine, releasing tension in the upper back. Blood circulation to the digestive organs is stimulated, which helps to regulate digestion. The shoulders and shoulder joints are also relaxed, increasing their suppleness.

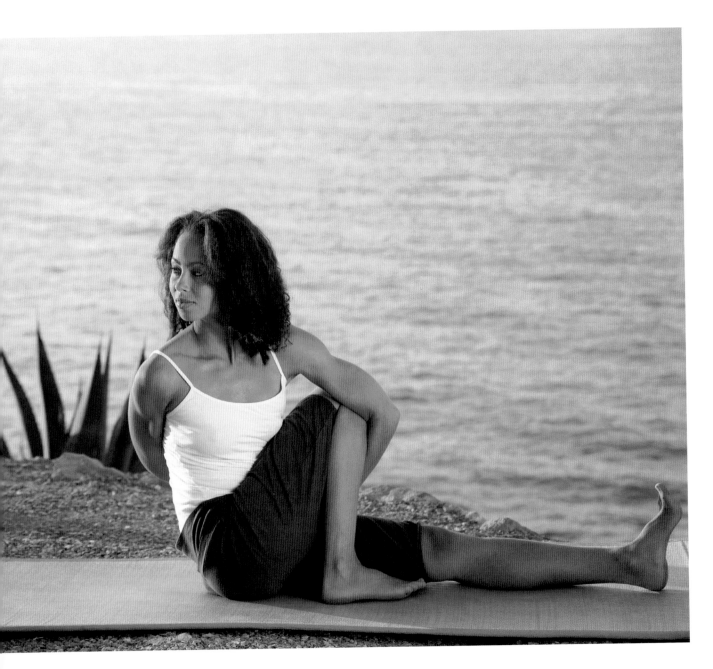

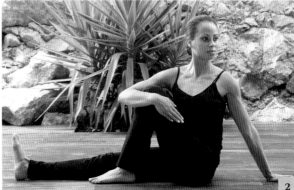

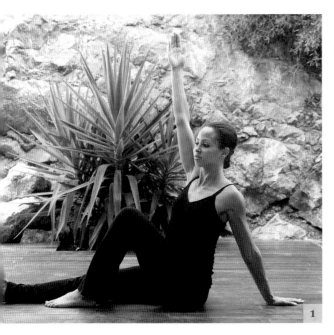

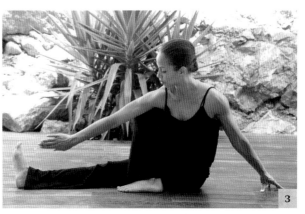

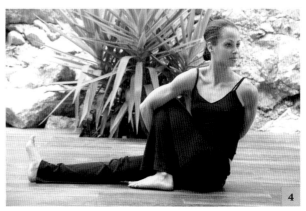

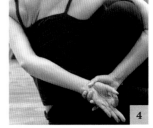

Step-by-step alignment

1. Sitting in an upright position, pull one leg up towards your chest. Keep the muscles of your outstretched leg taut. As you inhale, lengthen your spine through the crown of your head. Stretch the arm on the same side as your straight leg up towards the ceiling and place your other hand behind you.

2. As you exhale, twist to the side of your bent leg. Take your raised arm around your bent knee, drawing it gently in towards your body.

3. Maintain your breathing pattern and rotate the shoulder of your front arm inwards. Take this arm around the outer side of your bent knee and push this knee gently towards your body with your upper arm.

4. Now bend your front arm and extend it round the back of your body (see view from behind). Lift your other arm off the floor, take it behind your back and grasp the wrist with your other hand (see view from behind).

Each stage of the step-by-step alignment is good for practising. For the final stage, you can use a belt if you are not able to bring your hands together.

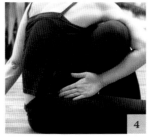

View from behind

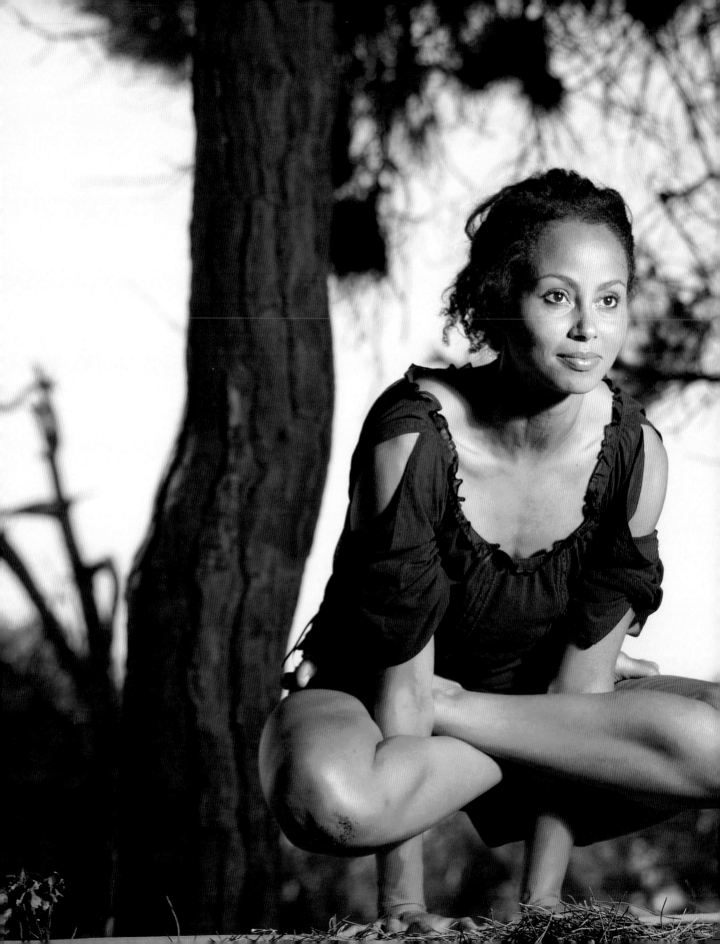

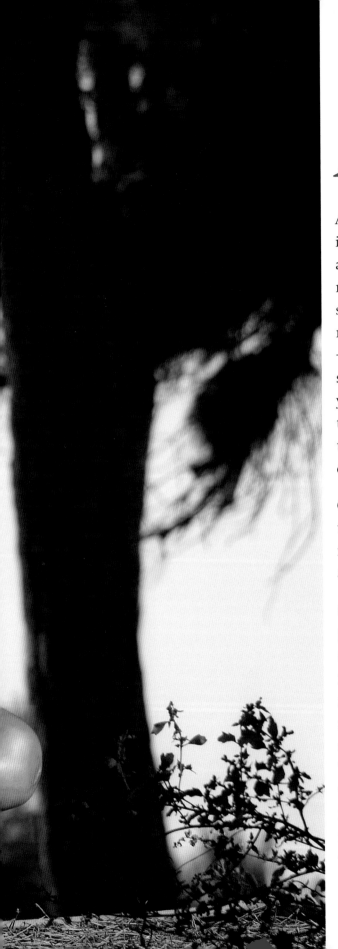

Arm balances

As the name implies, the arm balance positions involve balancing the body on the arms, and depend on finding and maintaining the moment between motion and stillness. Besides strength and practice, arm balances also require tremendous powers of concentration – and sometimes a fair degree of courage. Yoga students should note that practising specific yoga techniques (particularly performing the bandhas, see p.52) can, with time, help to channel the body's energy in a particular direction.

On a physical level, arm balances strengthen the arm, shoulder, back, stomach and leg muscles. They also energize the whole body and release vital energy.

On an emotional level, these asanas boost the powers of concentration, improve conscious awareness of the moment, and help to focus the body and mind. Arm balances also improve one's sense of balance and impart a feeling of equilibrium. They increase your self-confidence, because when you practise an arm balance, you are literally bearing all of your weight on your own arms. Some arm balances make you feel as if you are swaying, and you may experience an almost euphoric sense of weightlessness.

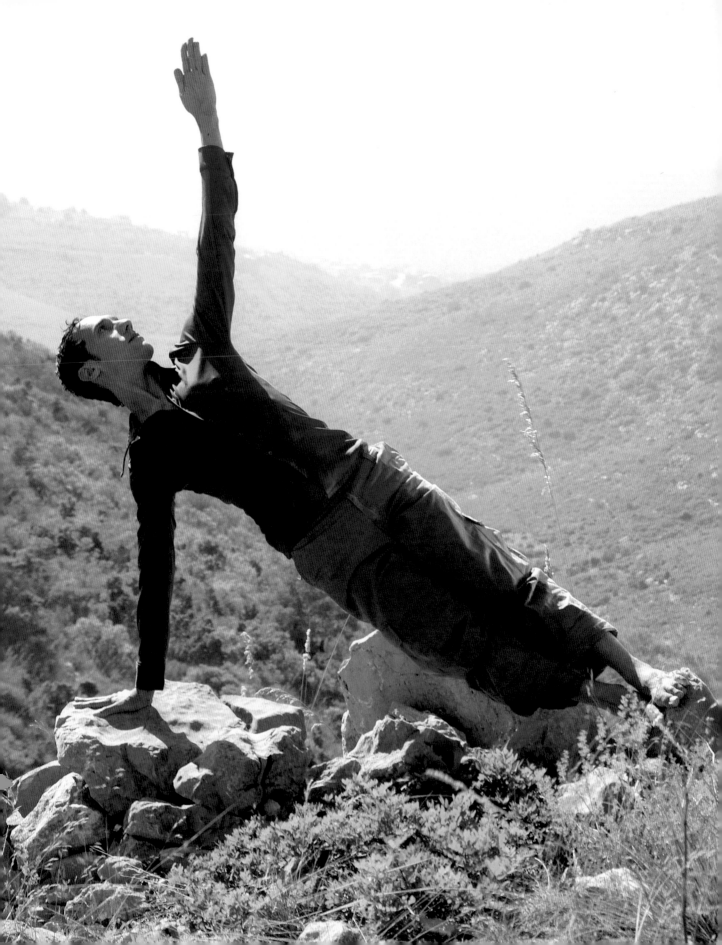

ᴠᴀsɪꜱᴛʜᴀꜱᴀɴᴀ Side Plank Pose

This asana strengthens the arms, the core and the leg muscles and invigorates the whole body, particularly the lumbar area, lumbar vertebrae and the tailbone. It also boosts the powers of concentration and ability to focus the mind, and improves the sense of balance.

Alignment

- Lie down on one side with the outer edge of your lower foot firmly on the floor and the insides of both feet directly next to each other.

- As you inhale, place your lower hand beneath your shoulder and lever yourself up from your shoulder.

- Form a straight line sideways with your body and push your hips up so that the core of your body does not sink towards the ground.

- As you exhale, raise your other arm into the air, so that both arms form a vertical line. Direct your gaze upwards.

- Keep the core of your body taut and stretch yourself out in all directions.

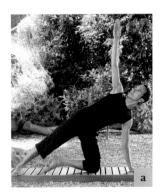
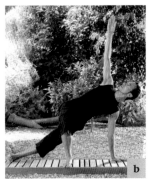

For beginners ▲

a. Rest your lower knee on the floor if you cannot hold your pelvis up. Form a straight line with your foot, lower knee and lower hand.

b. Alternatively, bend the knee of your upper leg and place your foot in front of you perpendicular to your pelvis; push this foot firmly into the ground.

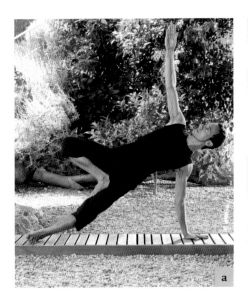

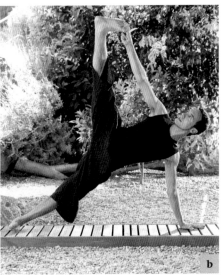

◄ **For advanced students**

a. Place the sole of your upper foot on the inside of the thigh of your lower leg.

b. Take hold of the big toe of your upper foot and draw this leg vertically into the air. Keep your hips open. This position is the full Vasisthasana.

Arm balances

बक़ासन bakasana   Crow Pose

Crow Pose tones the arm and stomach muscles, and strengthens the abdominal organs. It also boosts the powers of concentration, promotes inner focus and improves the sense of balance.

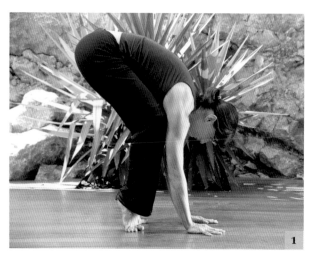

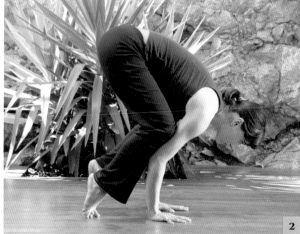

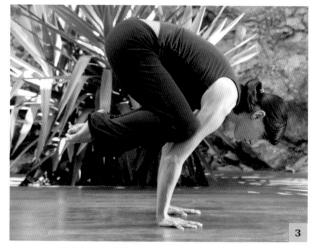

Step-by-step alignment

1. From a crouching position, rise up onto the tips of your toes. Bend forward and place your hands flat on the floor directly under your shoulders with your fingers spread wide apart. Push your buttocks up and draw your knees towards your armpits.

2. Round your back, place your knees on your upper arms, press your hands firmly into the ground and move your weight forward. Look as far in front of you as possible.

3. Tighten your stomach muscles, and as you inhale, perform Mula bandha (see p.52), raising your feet from the floor. As you exhale, perform Uddiyana bandha (see p.52) and push your buttocks up. Try to stretch your arms.

For beginners   ▶

Each individual stage of Bakasana is good for practising. If you cannot quite raise both legs from the floor at the same time in Step 3, practise lifting one leg at a time and keep your other foot on the floor to steady your balance.

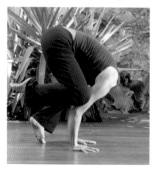

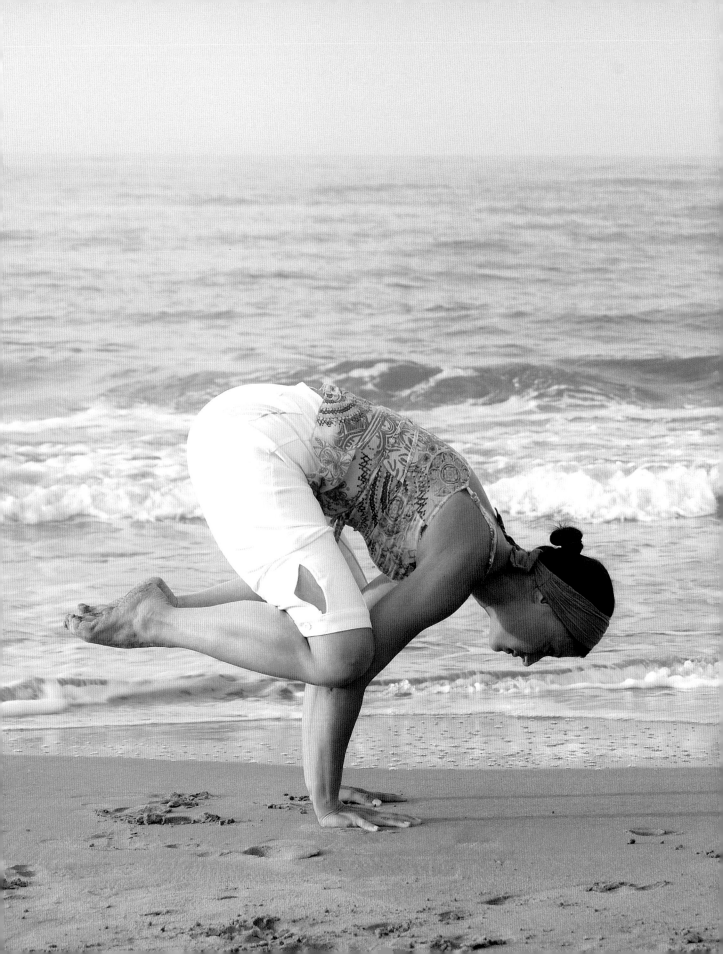

eka pada koundinyasana i
Pose dedicated to the sage Koundinya I

This asana strengthens the neck, arm and leg muscles. The pressure of the legs gives a gentle massage to the abdominal organs, while the twisting movement strengthens and energizes the spine. The posture also boosts the powers of concentration and promotes a sense of inner focus.

Step-by-step alignment

1. Get onto all fours and then move your hands slightly to the sides. Cross one leg over to the bent arm on the opposite side and rest this knee on your upper arm.

2. Look into the distance and shift your weight onto your hands, which should remain firmly pressed into the ground. Distribute your weight evenly over both hands. As you inhale, perform Mula bandha (see p.52) and raise both legs from the ground.

3. As you exhale, perform Uddiyana bandha (see p.52) and stretch both legs out: the back one backwards, and the one that is crossed to the side. Stretch forward through the crown of your head and back through your back leg.

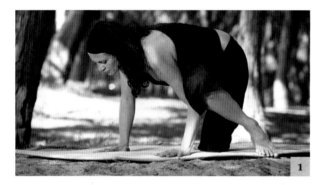

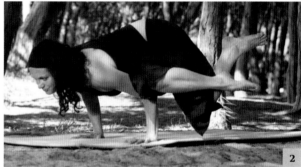

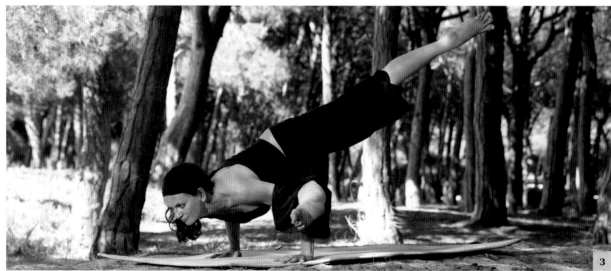

eka pada koundinyasana ii

Pose dedicated to the sage Koundinya II

This asana has the same beneficial effects as Eka Pada Koundinyasana I. It also provides an intense stretch to the muscles in the back of the thigh of the front leg.

Step-by-step alignment

1. Go onto all fours and stretch one leg out behind you. Bend your other leg over the bent arm on the same side.

2. Look straight ahead. As you inhale, perform Mula bandha (see p.52) and stretch your front leg out in front.

3. As you exhale, perform Uddiyana bandha (see p.52), shift your weight forward and raise your outstretched leg away from the floor behind you.

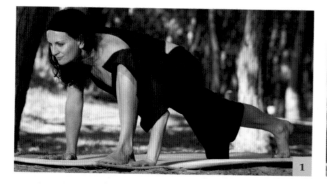

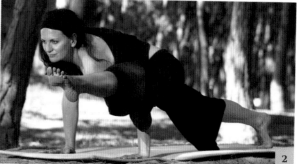

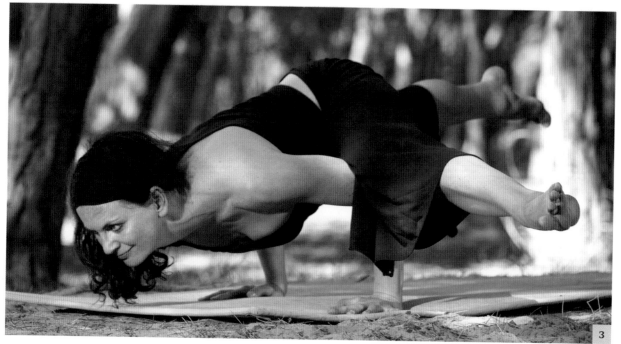

व्ह्स्वम्त्रस्वन Pose dedicated to the sage Visvamitra

This asana strengthens the arm, stomach and leg muscles. Besides requiring a great deal of strength in the arms and legs, it also demands the ability to stretch the thigh muscles and whole side of the body and also to open the hips wide. This posture improves the flexibility of the entire body.

Step-by-step alignment

1. Assume a sitting position, take your legs out to the side, and place your right hand flat on the floor beside your right thigh. Take hold of the outer edge of your right foot with your left hand and, bringing your right leg round the back of your arm, place it on your right upper arm near your shoulder.

2. As you inhale, stretch your right leg up behind your body.

3. Stretch out your right arm, rotate your shoulders outwards and, as you exhale, turn your upper body to the left.

4. Look at the ground to steady yourself, put pressure on your right hand and left foot, and tense your whole body. As you inhale, perform Mula bandha (see p.52) and raise your buttocks and both legs from the ground.

5. As you exhale, perform Uddiyana bandha (see p.52) and turn to the left again. Your weight should be distributed evenly over your left foot and right hand. Direct your gaze upwards. Repeat on the opposite side.

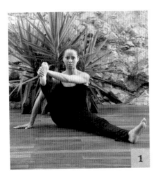

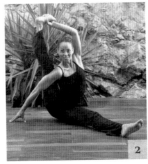

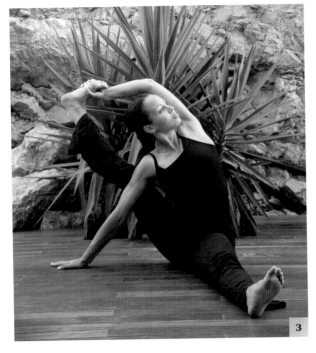

Visvamitrasana is a complex and challenging asana, which as well as a lot of practice also requires the muscles to be sufficiently warmed up and stretched. It is therefore important that you feel your way gently into this position by following the variations for beginners.

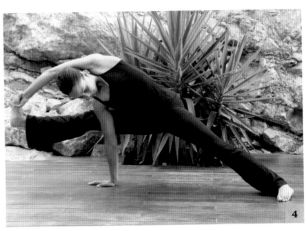

Arm balances

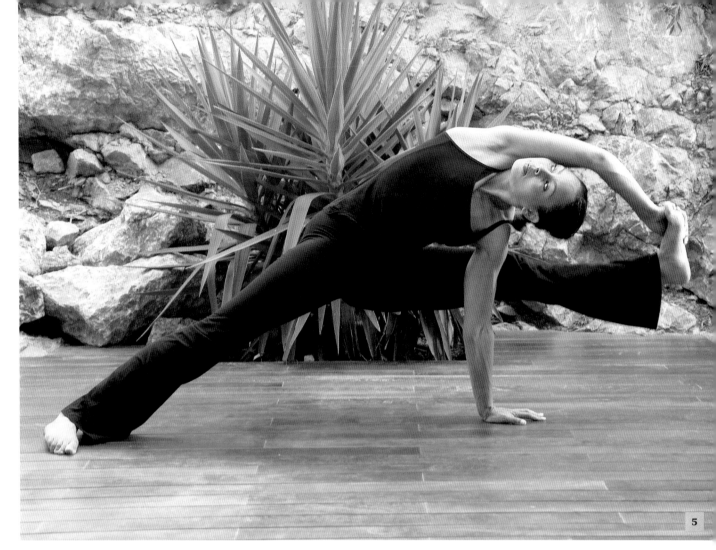

5

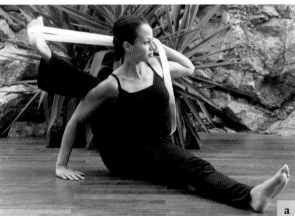

a

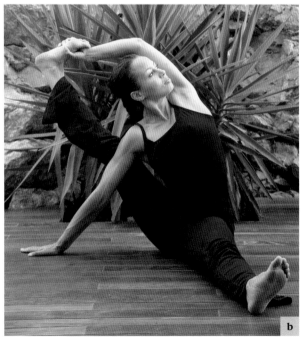

b

For beginners

a. Use a belt if you cannot reach your foot with your hand.

b. Practise up to Step 3 at first, until you can stay in this position for some time. This pose is called Konasana (corner) and is an asana in its own right.

bhujapidasana Shoulder Pressing Pose

This asana strengthens the arm, back and stomach muscles as well as the abdominal organs. It also boosts the powers of concentration and inner focus, and improves the sense of balance.

Step-by-step alignment

1. Sitting in a squat, spread your feet hip-width apart, lean forward and walk your hands back between your legs. Place your hands flat on the ground behind your feet and rest on your upper arms.

2. Look forward and shift your weight back. As you inhale, perform Mula bandha (see p.52) and raise both feet from the ground.

3. As you exhale, perform Uddiyana bandha (see p.52) and cross your feet in front of your upper body.

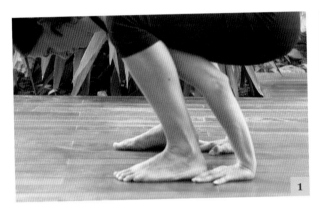

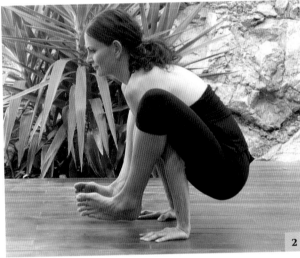

For beginners ▼

a. Place a block under each hand; this makes it easier to rest on your upper arms and lift your feet off the floor.

b. Try raising each foot from the ground in turn, while steadying yourself with your other foot.

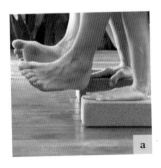

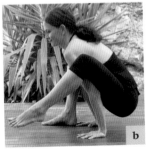

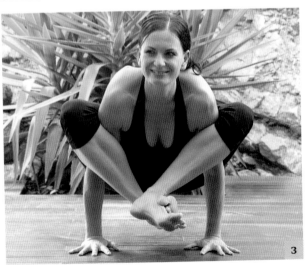

tittibhasana Firefly Pose

Firefly Pose strengthens the arm, back and stomach muscles as well as the abdominal organs. The spine is stretched, particularly from the lumbar vertebrae to the tailbone. It also boosts the powers of concentration and inner focus, and improves the sense of balance. As you practise this asana, you come to experience an almost euphoric feeling of lightness.

Alignment

- Follow the step-by-step alignment for Bhujapidasana up to Step 2 (see opposite).

- As you exhale, perform Uddiyana bandha (see p.52) and extend both legs straight or slightly raised in front of you.

Tittibhasana is a very challenging asana, so it is recommended that you practise Bhujapidasana first.

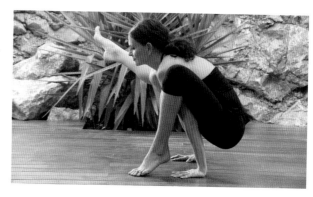

For beginners ▲

Try stretching each leg in front of you in turn, while steadying yourself with your other leg.

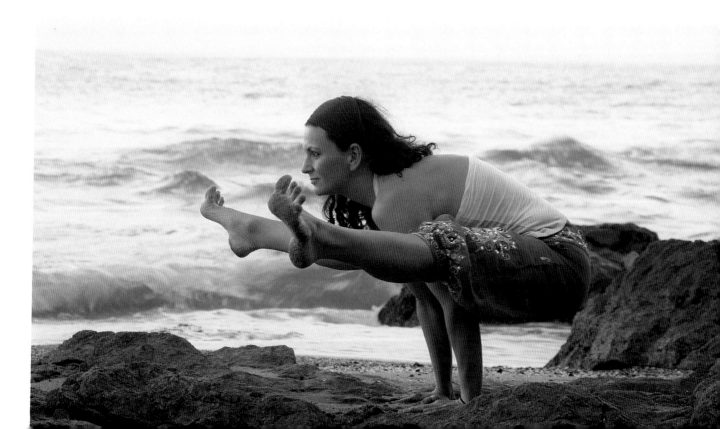

tolasana   Scale Pose

Scale Pose strengthens the arm, chest, back and stomach muscles. Padmasana (see p.206) also increases flexibility in the knee and foot muscles. In addition, it boosts the powers of concentration and the ability to focus. The sensation of hovering gives you a euphoric feeling of lightness.

Alignment

- Follow the step-by-step alignment for Padmasana (see p.206) to get into Lotus.

- Place both hands flat on the ground next to your hips, with the middle fingers facing forward. As you inhale, perform Mula bandha (see p.52), apply pressure on your hands and push yourself up.

- As you exhale, perform Uddiyana bandha (see p.52) and pull your crossed legs further up.

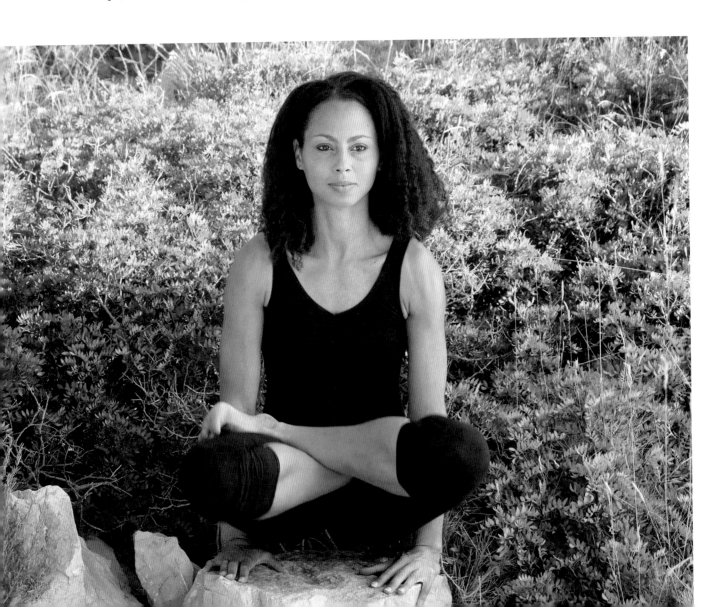

kukkutasana Cock Pose

Cock Pose has the same effect as Scale Pose. It also trains the sense of balance, because as you come out of the movement, you have to find your equilibrium.

Step-by-step alignment

1. Follow the step-by-step alignment for Padmasana (see p.206) to get into Lotus. Roll yourself onto your back in the Lotus position and put your upper arms between your thighs and calves. As you breathe in, perform Mula bandha (see p.52).

2. As you exhale, perform Uddiyana bandha (see p.52) and roll yourself forward.

3. Put your hands flat on the floor, shift your weight forward, and find the moment at which your whole body is resting on your hands and you are balanced.

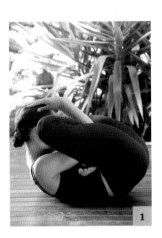
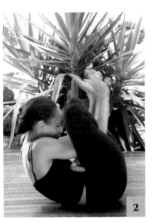
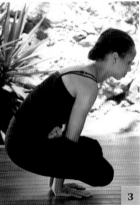
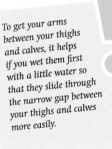

Side view

To get your arms between your thighs and calves, it helps if you wet them first with a little water so that they slide through the narrow gap between your thighs and calves more easily.

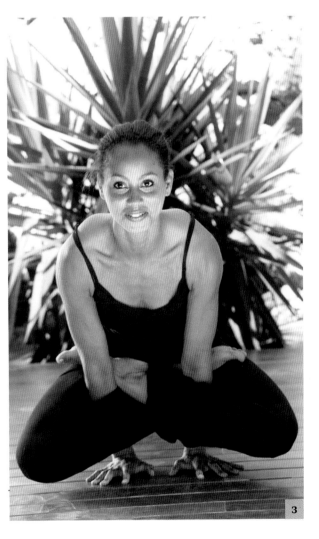

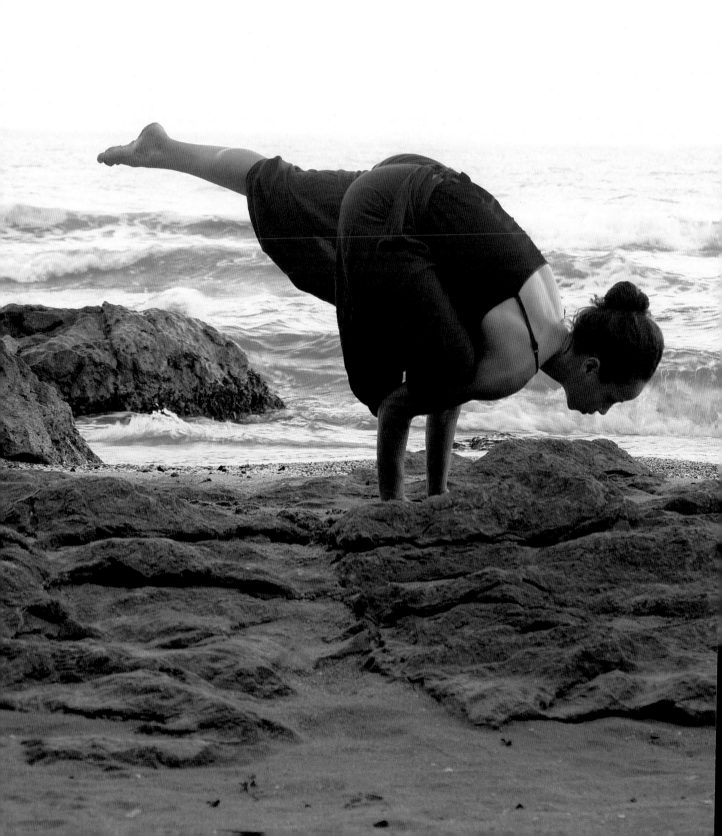

एका पादा गालवासन (eka pada galavasana)   **Flying Crow Pose**

Flying Crow Pose strengthens the whole body: the hand, arm, shoulder, chest, back, stomach, buttock and leg muscles. At the same time, the abdominal organs are massaged. This asana also challenges the sense of balance and powers of concentration, and gives a feeling of levity: the sense of flying.

Step-by-step alignment

1. From a standing position, bend both legs and place the shin bone of one leg on the knee of the other. Put your palms together.

2. Place your hands on the floor in front of you and press the foot of the crossed-over leg against your upper arm (see detailed view).

3. Look into the distance, and as you inhale, perform Mula bandha (see p.52), shift your weight forward onto your hands and raise your back leg from the ground.

4. As you exhale, perform Uddiyana bandha (see p.52), push your bottom up and stretch your back leg out.

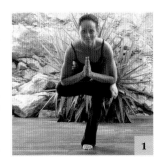

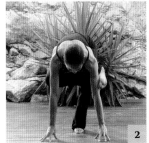

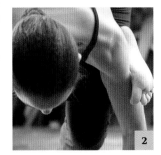

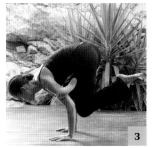

Detailed view

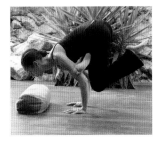

For beginners ▲

If you are a little afraid of shifting your weight forward, place a cushion under your face.

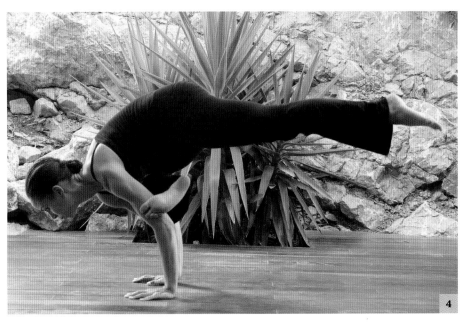

eka hasta bhujasana   Leg over Arm Balance

This asana strengthens the whole body: the hand, arm, shoulder, chest, back, stomach, buttock and leg muscles. At the same time, the abdominal organs are massaged. It also challenges the sense of balance and the powers of concentration.

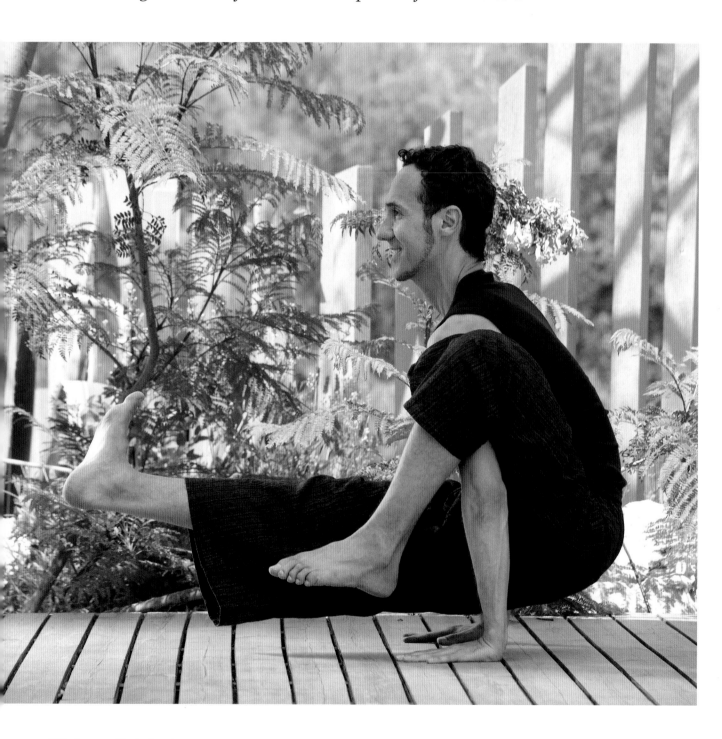

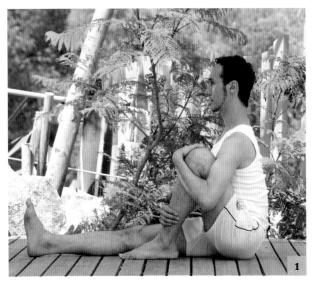

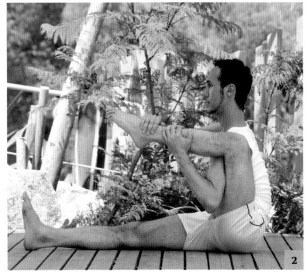

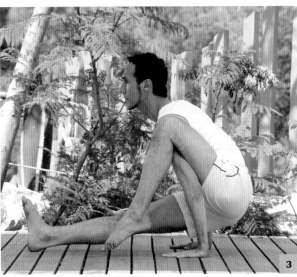

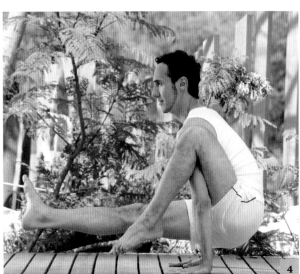

Step-by-step alignment

1. Sit on the floor with your pelvis level and bring one leg up to your chest.

2. Bring the thigh of your bent leg up round the back of the upper arm towards your shoulder.

3. Place the palms of your hands flat on the floor beside your hips and look straight ahead. As you inhale, perform Mula bandha (see p.52), press your hands firmly into the floor and lift your bottom up from the ground. Stretch yourself up through the crown of your head.

4. As you exhale, perform Uddiyana bandha (see p.52) and raise your outstretched leg from the floor. Push the heel of the foot of your straight leg firmly away from you.

Each individual stage is good for practising on its own.

अष्टावक्रासन ashtavakrasana   Pose dedicated to the sage Ashtavakra

This asana strengthens the arm, shoulder, chest, stomach, buttock and leg muscles. At the same time, the abdominal organs are massaged by the contraction of the upper body. The sense of balance and powers of concentration are also challenged.

Arm balances

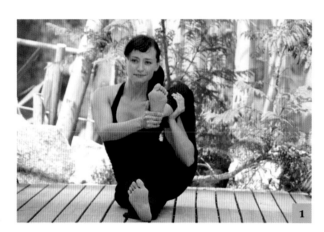

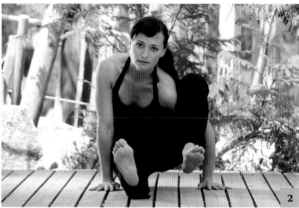

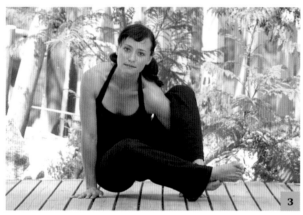

Step-by-step alignment

1. Sit on the floor with your pelvis level, bring one leg up to your chest and take the thigh of your bent leg up around the back of your upper arm towards your shoulder.

2. Place the palms of your hands flat on the floor beside your hips and look to the front. As you inhale, perform Mula bandha (see p.52), press your hands firmly into the floor and raise your bottom and your outstretched leg from the ground.

3. As you exhale, cross your feet. On the next inhalation, shift your weight gently forward and swivel your legs to the side of your bent leg.

4. As you exhale, perform Uddiyana bandha (see p.52) and stretch both legs out to the side.

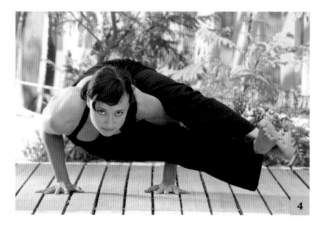

Each individual stage is good for practising on its own. However, the main prerequisites for performing complex asanas like this are patience and calm.

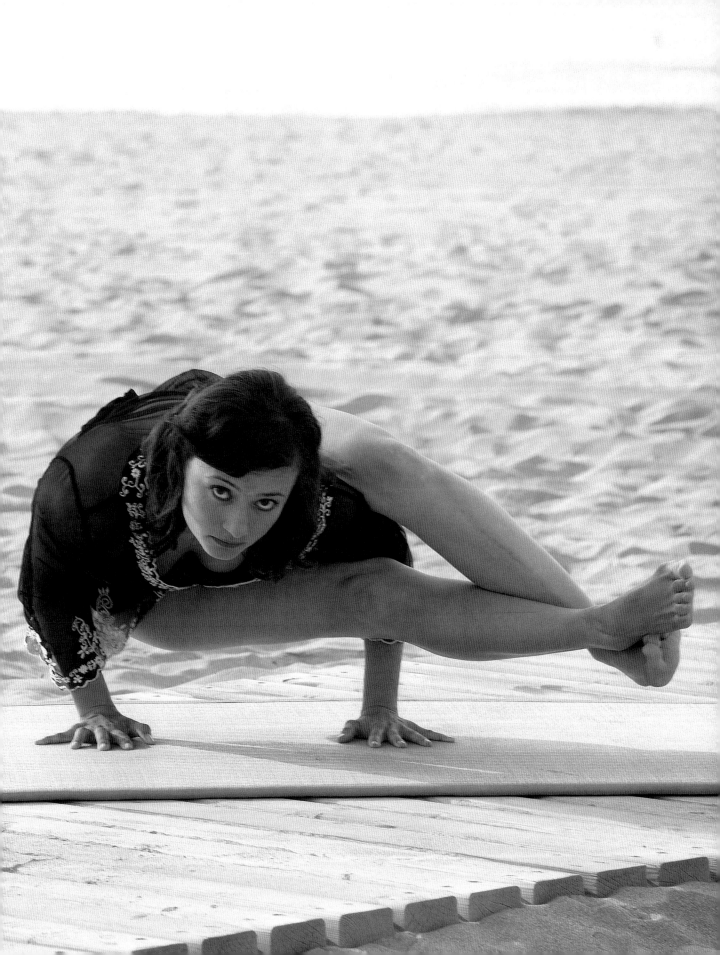

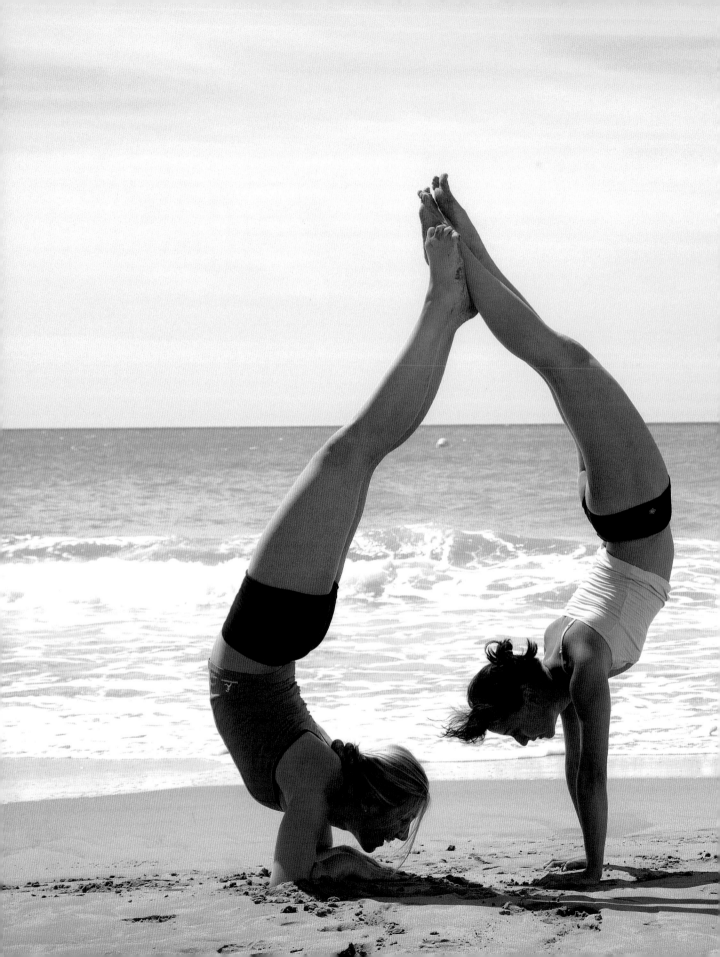

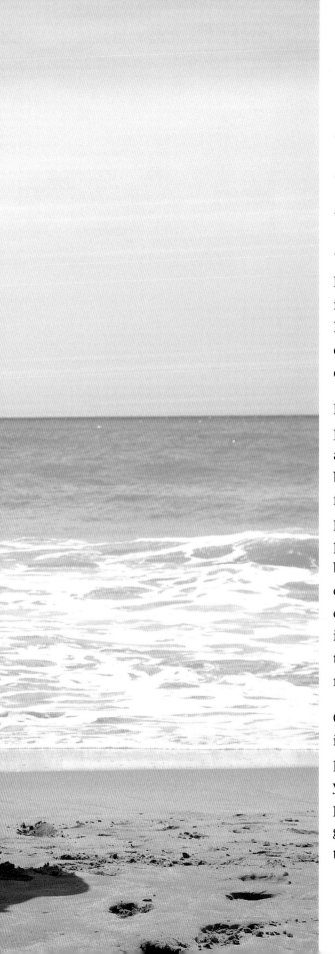

Inverted postures

In inverted yoga poses the natural body posture is literally turned on its head. The shoulders, head, arms or hands become bearers of their own weight – a beneficial but challenging experience.

From a physiological point of view, inverted postures stimulate the blood circulation around the whole body, particularly to the brain, lymphs and glands. Pressure is relieved from the legs, all of the body's organs and particularly the heart. Some of these inverted postures require a lot of practice, strength and body tension. But if you consider that they can promise eternal youth and beauty, the effort is well worth it. Care should be taken if you suffer from high blood pressure, and these poses should not be practised during menstruation, or if you have neck problems.

On an emotional level, inverted postures impart a feeling of stability and balance, peace and calm, even when the world around you is in turmoil. They also give you a new perspective on life. This is why they can often give you the courage to overcome fears and the strength to start something new.

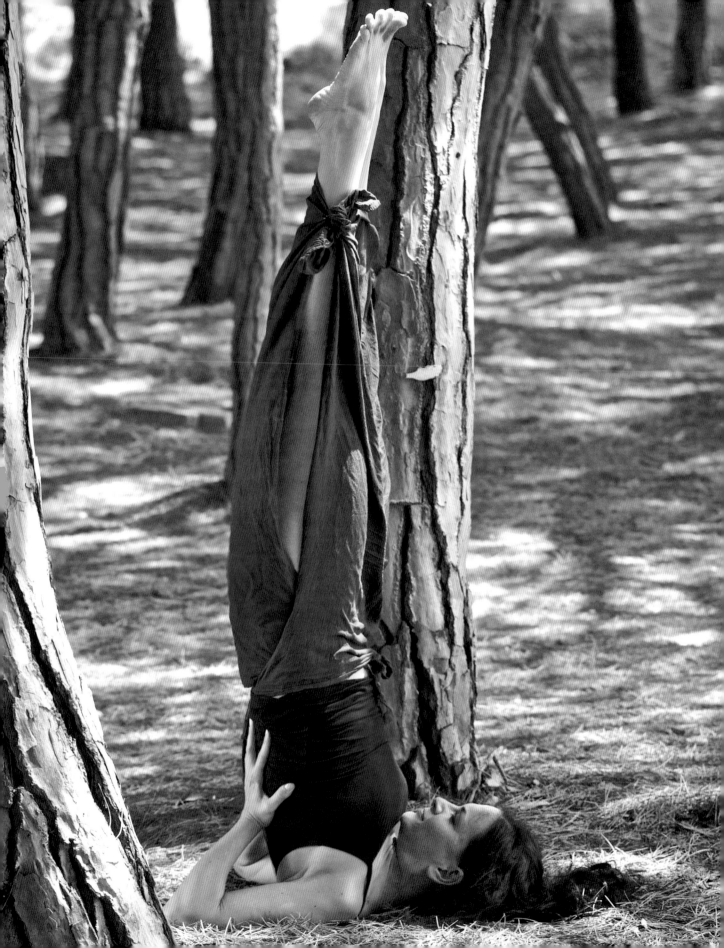

ṣālambā ṣārvangāṣānā Supported Shoulder Stand

This asana is also called the 'Mother of all Asanas', because it has a variety of positive effects. The blood circulation is stimulated, and the legs and organs are relieved and relaxed. The airways are cleared and the hormonal balance stimulated. In short, this posture gives new energy, confidence and strength.

Alignment

- It is easiest to come out of Halasana (see p.186) into a shoulder stand. Bring your elbows as close together as possible and support your back with your hands; your fingertips should be pointing straight up.

- As you inhale, stretch one leg up, followed by the other.

- As you exhale, stretch your whole body up through to your feet and push your tailbone towards your heels. Keep your back as straight as possible.

- Your gaze should be directed up towards your legs. Do not move your head. Keep on stretching yourself upwards and do not let yourself sink down.

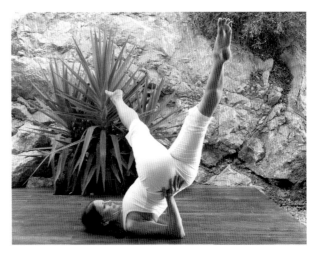

Variation ▲

Support your sacrum with a flat hand, rotate through your lower spine to the side and allow your pelvis to sink onto your hand – this results in a combination of an inverted posture and a twist. If you want to, you can try straddling your legs.

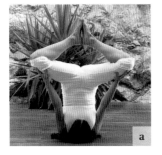
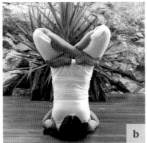

a   b

For advanced students ▲

a. Bend your legs and put the soles of your feet together. Stretch your arms up and steady your knees with your hands. Make sure you keep your weight on your shoulders.

b. Fold your legs in Padmasana (see p. 206). Support your back with one hand if you need the other to get into the Padmasana position.

Take care with neck problems, high blood pressure and during menstruation. Rest your legs against a wall, or feel yourself gently into this position. Observe how your body feels after practising this shoulder stand.

ह‌ालासन halasana   The Plough

This asana gives you the same benefits as Salamba Sarvangasana (see pp.184–5). The abdominal organs are also stimulated by the pressure of the legs, and the stretch in the shoulders is increased. 'Hal' means 'poison', and this asana is reputed to expel 'poison' from the throat, thus promoting better communication.

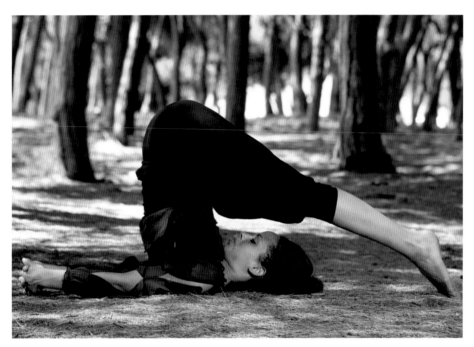

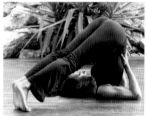

Variation: Parsva Halasana, Side Plough Pose ▲

Support your back with your hands, rotate your spine to one side and bring your closed legs to the same side. This results in a combination of an inverted posture and a twist.

Alignment

- Lie flat on your back and bend one leg.

- Take hold of the knee of your bent leg, and as you inhale, swing both legs over behind your head.

- If possible, stretch out your legs as you exhale, put your toes on the ground, make your back as flat as possible and pull your pubic bone up.

- Stretch your arms out and fold your hands. Put pressure on your arms and bring your shoulders under your body as far as you can.

- Make sure that your weight is being carried by your shoulders. The neck should remain relaxed and long. Place a blanket under your shoulders if your neck does not feel relaxed.

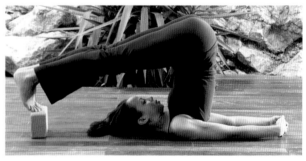

For beginners ▲

Place a block under your feet if you cannot quite reach the floor with your legs outstretched.

Take care with neck problems, high blood pressure and during menstruation. Rest your legs against a wall, or feel yourself gently into the position. Observe how your body feels after practising this posture. This also applies to Karnapidasana (see opposite).

karnapidasana Knee to Ear Pose

This is a good position to rest in – the whole torso, particularly the heart, and the legs can relax. The gentle arching of the back stretches the spine and stimulates the abdominal organs. You almost get a feeling of retreating to an inner island, as closing the ears and eyes shuts out all external stimuli.

Alignment

- Assume the Halasana position (see opposite). As you exhale, bend your knees and draw them up to your ears.

- As you inhale, take your arms back and grab hold of the wrist of one hand with the other hand. Keep your back as upright as possible.

If you cannot get your knees either side of your ears, just bring them to your forehead.

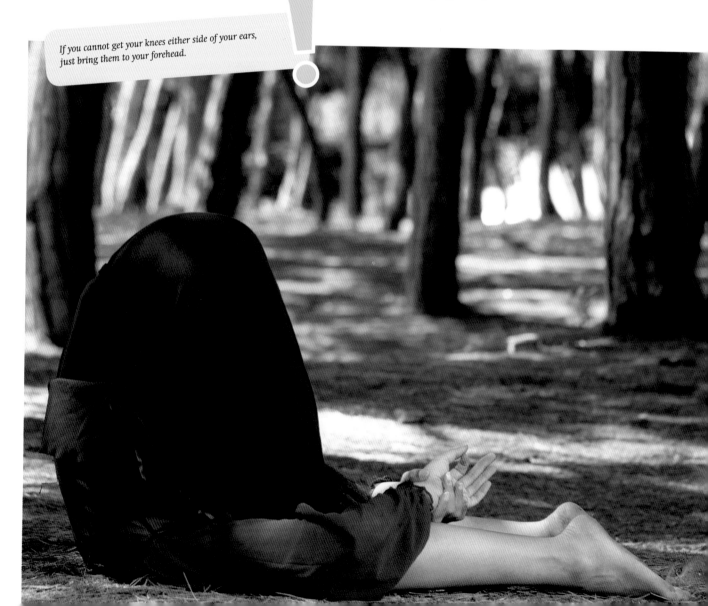

ṣalamba ṣhirṣhaṣana i Supported Headstand I

Supported Headstand I is also called the 'Queen of the Asanas', because, like Salamba Sarvangasana (see pp.184–5), it has a variety of positive effects. Blood circulation, particularly to the brain, lymphs and glands, is stimulated. The effects of gravity bring relief and relaxation to the legs and organs. The airways are cleared and hormonal balance is stimulated. The act of balancing conveys a sense of stability and equilibrium, and increases feelings of self-confidence.

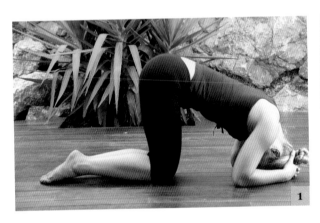

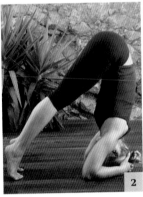

Practise Steps 1 and 2 until you can get your pelvis above your body and your legs rise up almost by themselves.

Step-by-step alignment

1. Starting on all fours, lower your forearms down to the ground shoulder-width apart. Fold your hands (with the little fingers one above the other) to form a 'basket' for your head. Put the crown of your head on the ground and steady your head with your hands.

2. Stretch your legs and walk your feet towards your body until your pelvis is almost above your shoulders. Support most of your weight on your forearms – not on your head – and push upwards from your shoulders.

3. As you inhale, take one leg up, followed by the other – either outstretched or bent. When your pelvis is above your body, your legs will go up almost by themselves. Never use force to jump into a headstand!

4. As you exhale, press your heels up and push your tailbone up too. Your whole body should be working, particularly your core. Make

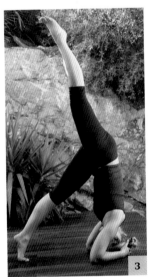

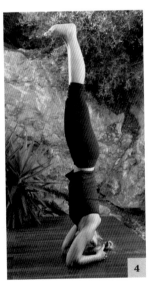

sure that your weight is carried by your forearms and that you do not sink into your shoulders.

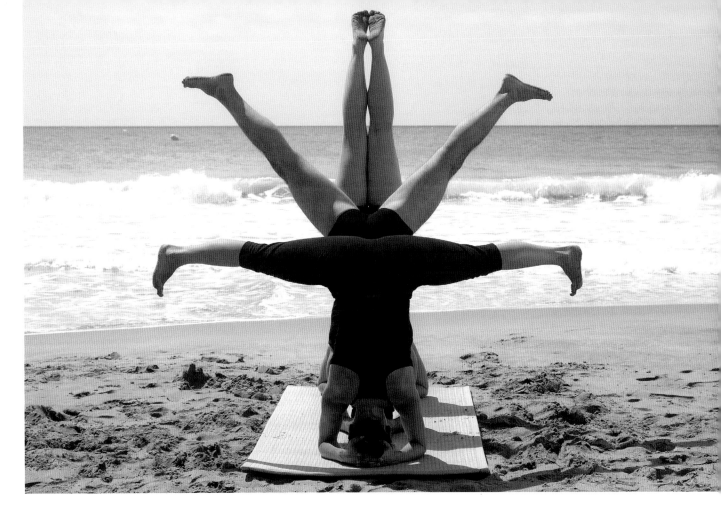

Variation: Salamba Shirshasana II ▼ ▶

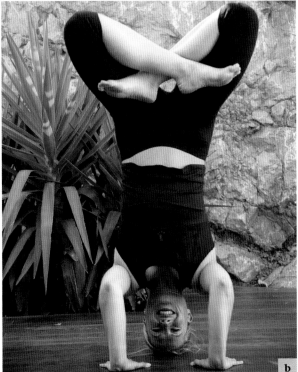

a. Splay your fingers out and place your hands and the crown of your head on the floor to form a triangle. Continue by following Steps 1–4. If you are not steady enough yet to stretch your legs out straight above you, rest your knees on your upper arms to help you develop a feeling of balance.

b. The headstand in Padmasana (see p.206). This is a special kind of challenge that is only recommended after you have mastered the headstand and should only be practised on a very firm surface. Come into Padmasana, swing yourself onto your knees and follow the instructions given in Variation (a).

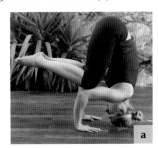

Take care with neck problems, high blood pressure and during menstruation. Rest your legs against a wall, or feel yourself gently into the position. Observe how you feel after practising this posture.

pincha mayurasana Forearm Stand

Besides the general beneficial effects of inverted postures, this asana also strengthens the shoulders and arms. In addition, it has the same positive effects of a backbend (see pp.122–43). In short, this position provides you with strength, confidence and self-assurance – although at first it may present something of a challenge to master.

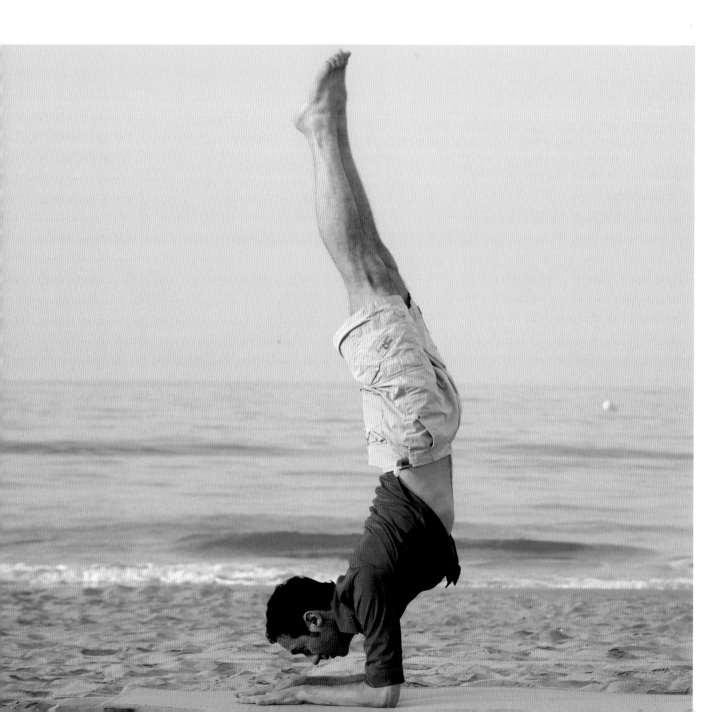

Step-by-step alignment

1. Come into Adho Mukha Svanasana (see p.67). Lower your forearms to the ground, positioning your elbows in a parallel line directly below your shoulders and stretching your forearms out straight. Your fingers should be splayed open as in Adho Mukha Svanasana. Look straight ahead.

2. Shift your weight onto your forearms and push up through your shoulders. Raise one leg.

3. As you inhale, perform Mula bandha (see p.52) and swing both legs up, pushing your breastbone forward and lengthening yourself from your thoracic vertebrae.

4. Practise against a wall first, so that when both legs are outstretched you can place your feet against the wall to support yourself.

5. As you exhale, push up through your shoulders again and then either take one foot away at a time or both feet away from the wall at once. As you do so, perform Uddiyana bandha (see p.52) and steady your core by pushing your tailbone up.

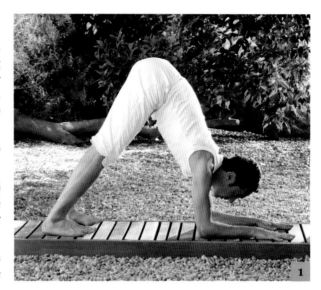

1

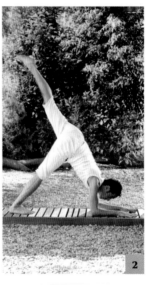

2

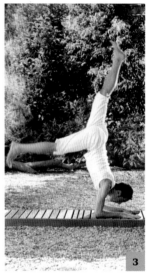

3

Pinchya Mayurasana is a complex position for which you should prepare with gentle backbends (see pp.122–43). You should also have sufficient strength in your arms and lots of flexibility in your shoulders, which you can build up with Adho Mukha Svanasana (see p.67) and Chatturanga Dandasana (see pp.68–9).

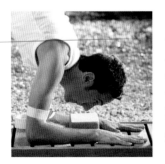

◀ **For beginners**

To prevent the position of your arms from changing, tie a belt around your upper arms and/or place a block between your forearms.

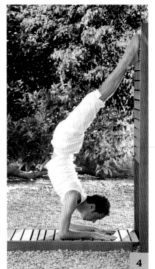

4

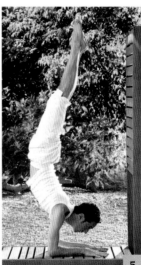

5

adho mukha vrikshasana Handstand

Besides the general beneficial effects of inverted postures (see pp.182–93) and backbends (see pp.122–43), this asana strengthens the shoulders, arms and wrists. The Handstand also gives strength, confidence and self-assurance – even though it does take quite a lot of effort to master.

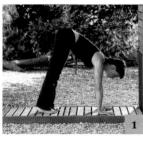
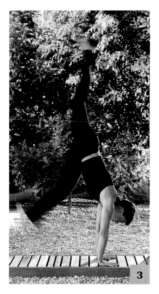
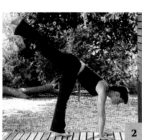
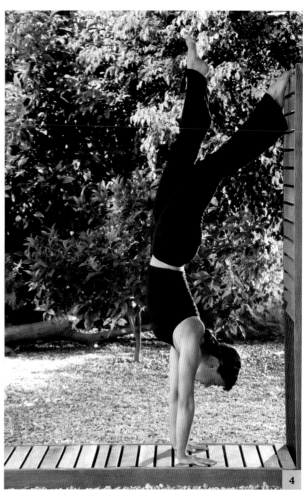

Step-by-step alignment

1. Bend forward from a standing position and place your wrists directly below your shoulders. Splay out your fingers to enable you to put weight on the whole hand. Look to the front.

2. Shift your weight onto your hands and with straight arms push up through your shoulders. Raise one leg.

3. As you inhale, perform Mula bandha (see p.52) and swing both legs up, pushing your breastbone forward and lengthening yourself from your thoracic vertebrae.

Adho Mukha Vrikshasana is a complex position for which you should prepare with gentle backbends (see pp.122–43). You should also have sufficient strength in your arms and lots of flexibility in your shoulders, which you can build up with Adho Mukha Svanasana (see p.67) and Chatturanga Dandasana (see pp.68–9.).

4. Practise against a wall first, so that when both legs are outstretched you can place your feet against the wall to support yourself. As you exhale, push up through your shoulders again and then either take one foot away from the wall at a time or both feet away from the wall simultaneously. As you do so, perform Uddiyana bandha (see p.52) and steady your core by pushing your tailbone up.

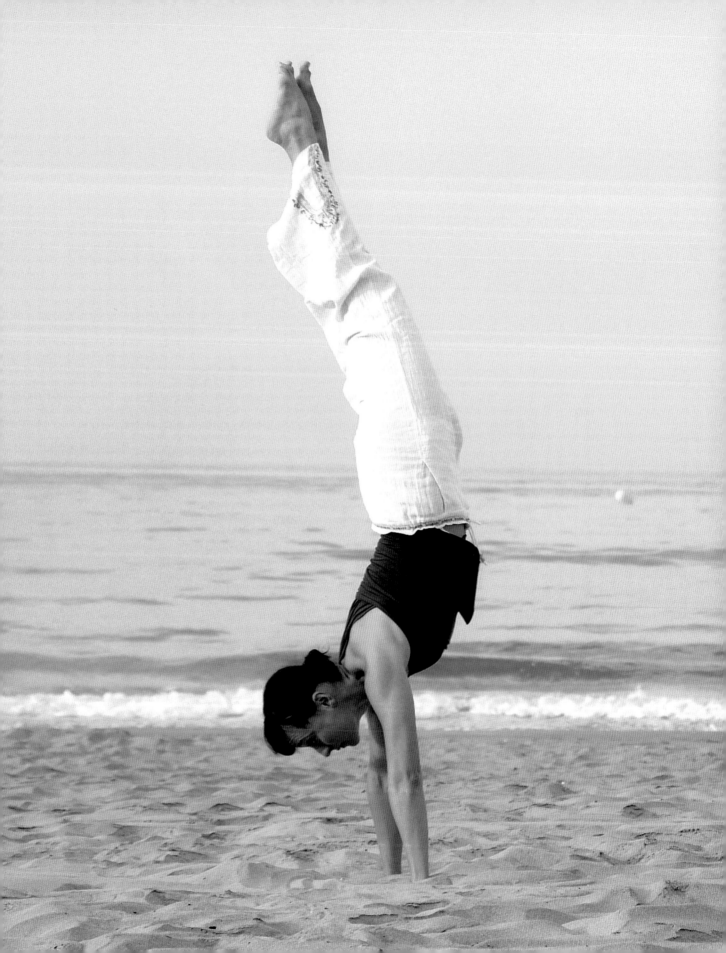

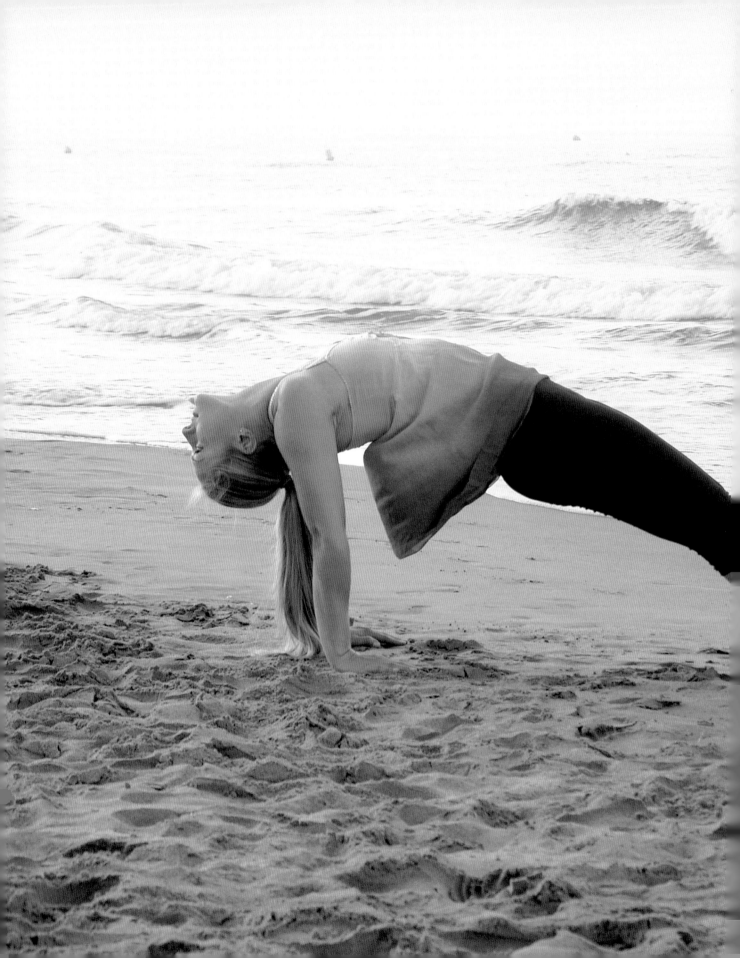

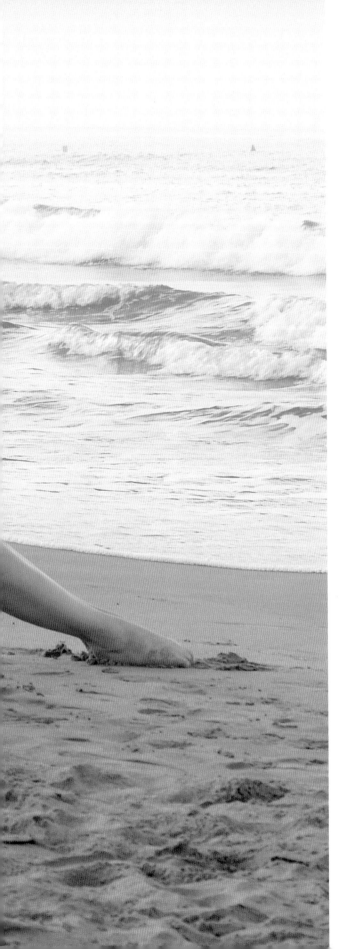

Neutral postures

In the following asanas the spine remains neutral, hence the name 'neutral postures'. Some are mainly suitable as balancing postures after forward and backward bends, while others also provide good meditating positions, which are practised with a straight spine in an upright position.

From a physiological point of view, most neutral floor postures stretch the spine and reduce stiffness in the knees and ankles. They also open up the hips and lumbar area, giving the body the strength and flexibility required for longer meditations.

On an emotional level, neutral asanas have a calming and balancing effect. The spirit can find peace and the poses make it easier to shut out external distractions that can divert the mind.

ᛗalasana **Squat Pose**

In this position, the hips are opened wide and the calf muscles are given an intense stretch. The lengthening of the spine enables the whole back to relax, alleviating tension in this area.

Alignment

- Crouch down on the balls of your feet, placing your feet hip-width apart.
- Gently lower your heels to the floor, allow your buttocks to sink further and push your tailbone down.
- Place the palms of your hands together and press your upper arms gently against your knees to steady yourself and open your hips further.

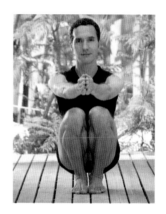

◄ Variation

Practise the squat with your knees together. Although your hips remain closed in this pose, your spine is given an added stretch. This variation also trains your sense of balance.

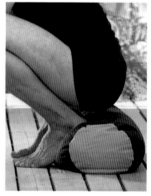

For beginners ▲

Place a cushion under your heels if you are unable to lower them to the floor.

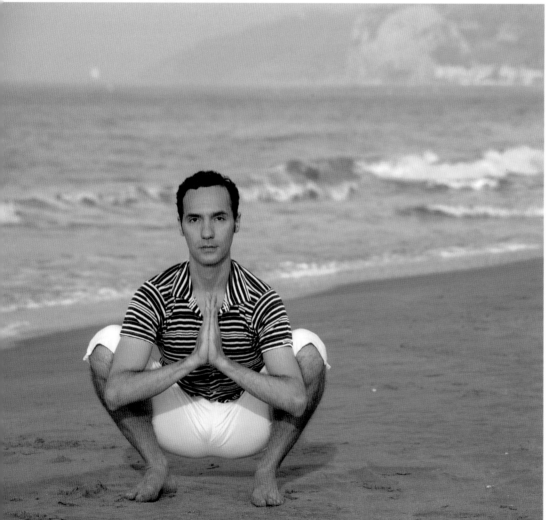

purvottanasana Upward Plank Pose

In this asana, the whole front of the body is stretched. The wrists and ankles are strengthened, and the shoulders and chest area are opened wide. Raising the pelvis stabilizes and stretches the spine.

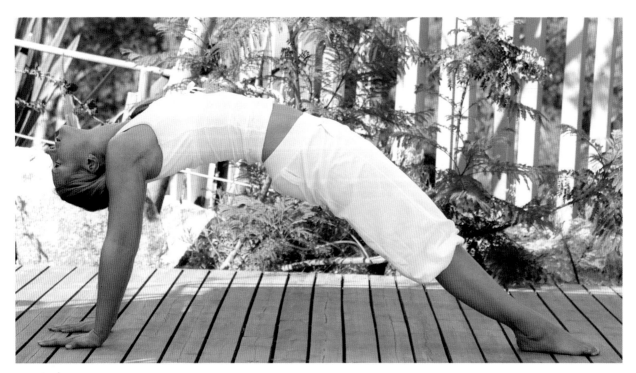

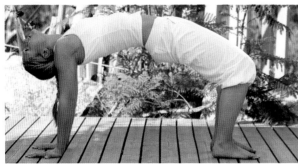

For beginners ▲

If you are unable to stretch your legs out comfortably, bend them to a right angle, making sure that you keep your knees directly over your ankles. Because of the shape the body makes, this position is also called 'Table Pose'.

Alignment

- Sit on the floor with your legs stretched out and your hands about a hand's width behind your bottom; your fingers can point forward or backward (but not to the side).

- As you inhale, push down through your hands and feet, and raise your pelvis and legs from the ground, keeping the soles of your feet flat on the floor.

- As you exhale, stretch out, pushing your tailbone down towards your feet and resting your head on your shoulder muscles, provided that you do not suffer from neck problems.

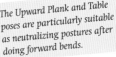

The Upward Plank and Table poses are particularly suitable as neutralizing postures after doing forward bends.

dandasana Staff Pose

This posture gives a stretch to the whole spine and the muscles at the back of the thighs. It is a good position for neutralizing the spine following gentle forward or backward bends.

Alignment

- Sit upright on the floor with your legs outstretched and place the palms of your hands next to your hips. Keep your pelvis level.

- Tense the muscles in your legs, pull your toes towards your body and push your heels away. Apply pressure to your hands, and as you inhale, lengthen your spine, pulling up through the crown of your head.

- Relax and, as you exhale, open your shoulders and push your tailbone down. Maintain the length in your spine.

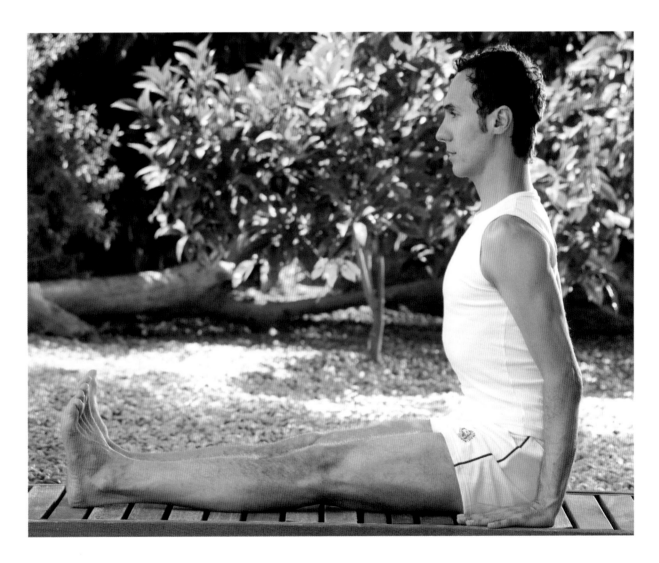

सिंहासन Simhasana   Lion Pose

Lion Pose helps to relieve bad breath and release tension, particularly in the face and jaw muscles. This position is good for learning to let go; one of the reasons for this is that, as you practise the Lion, you learn to lose all inhibitions and feelings of embarrassment at looking a little strange.

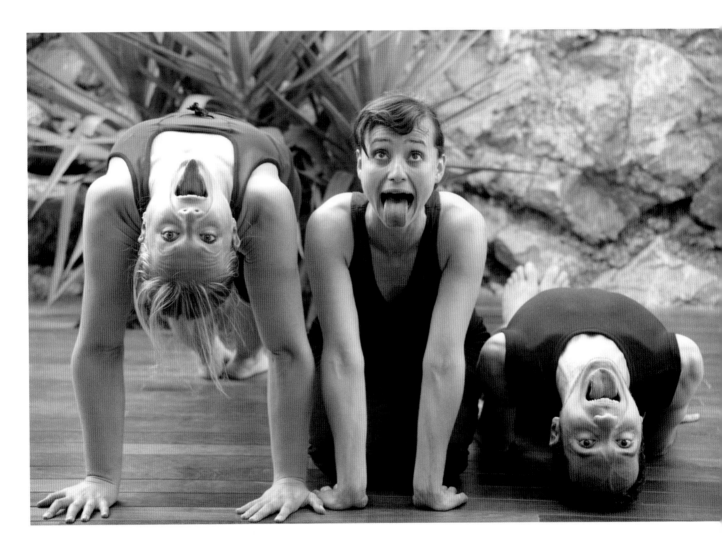

Alignment

- Traditionally Simhasana is practised in Vajrasana with straightened arms (see p.205), or in Purvottanasana (see p.197) or Matsyasana (see p.137).

- Take a deep breath. Then breathe out making a loud hissing noise, and stick your tongue out as far as possible (pointing the tip of your tongue towards your chin). Focus on your 'third eye', i.e. the point between your eyebrows.

> Simhasana can be done in any asana, but is generally practised in the postures mentioned here.

ꞯꞯꞯꞯꞯ navaṣana Boat Pose

This position stretches the whole of the spine, and strengthens the lower back and the stomach and leg muscles. The tensioning of the abdominal muscles helps to ease feelings of fullness and any gastro-intestinal discomfort. The posture also sharpens the sense of balance.

Alignment

- Move into Dandasana (see p.198). As you inhale, perform Mula bandha (see p.52) and stretch your outstretched legs up until your body forms a 'V' shape. At the same time, stretch your arms out towards your knees.

- As you exhale, perform Uddiyana bandha (see p.52) and push your tailbone down. Maintain the length in your spine and keep your balance on your bottom.

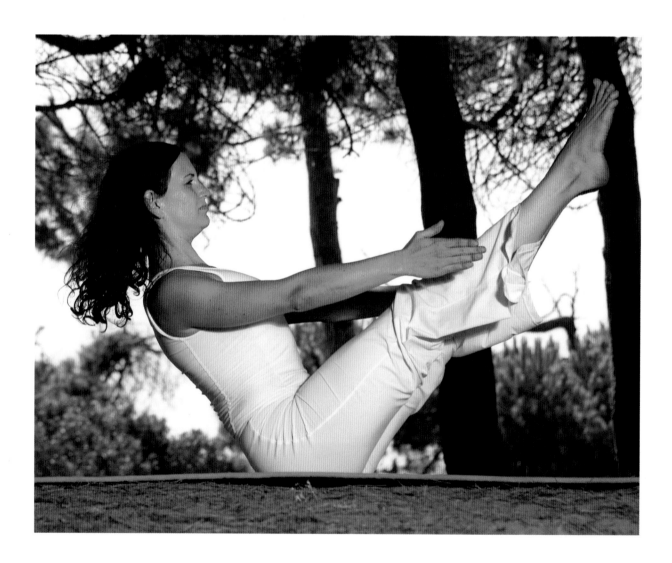

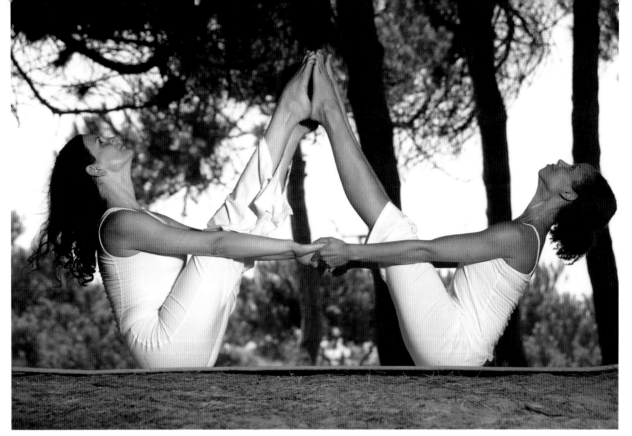

Navasana as a paired asana

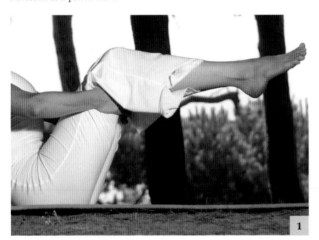

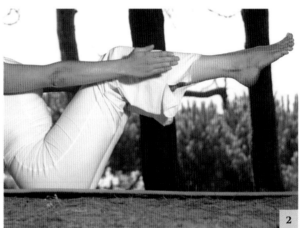

For beginners ▲

1. If you have difficulty maintaining a straight back and keeping upright with your legs outstretched, and find yourself tipping backwards, bend your legs and steady yourself by holding onto the backs of your knees.

2. Let go of your knees and try to keep your balance.

Navasana requires strong stomach muscles to be able to maintain a straight back. If your stomach muscles are not quite strong enough to keep you balanced, try bending your legs.

ꢱukhaꢱana Easy Pose

In this posture, the spine is kept straight and stretched, and the hips are gently opened. The body is centred and calmed. This makes the pose suitable for switching off for a short time, allowing you to gather your thoughts, concentrate or meditate. It also makes a good starting position for a yoga class.

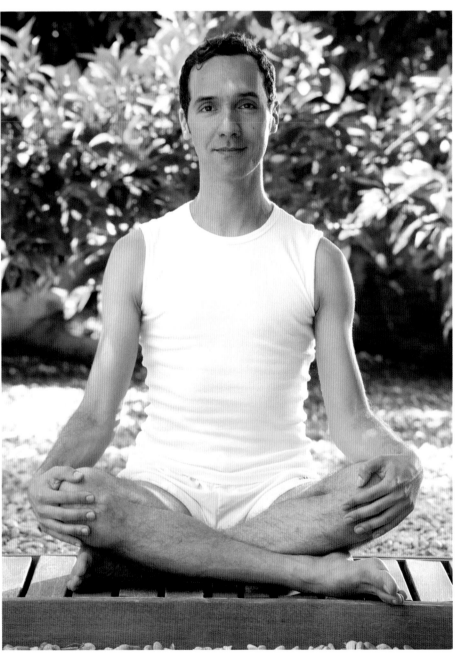

Alignment

- Sit on the floor with your back straight and your legs crossed. Allow your sit bones, hips and knees to sink to the floor.

- Straighten your spine and pull up through the crown of your head. Keep your back straight, particularly at the base.

- Place your hands in a relaxed position on your knees or thighs. Look into the distance or close your eyes.

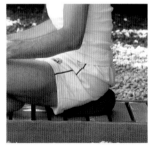

For beginners ▲

Sit on a cushion if you cannot sit straight comfortably.

siddhasana/muktasana **Perfect Pose**

This position is very similar to Sukhasana (opposite), but is a little harder because it demands a certain amount of flexibility in the hips and knees. In this asana the body remains centred and calm, making it one of the classic meditation poses. However, it can also be used to switch off for a short time, allowing you to gather your thoughts and concentrate.

Alignment

- Sit on the floor and bend one leg. Bring the heel of your bent leg as close to your pubic bone as possible. Bend your other leg and place the heel directly in front of the other one.

- Allow your sit bones, hips and knees to sink to the floor.

- Straighten your spine and pull up through the crown of your head. Keep your back straight, particularly at the base.

- Place your hands in a relaxed position on your knees or in your lap, and look into the distance or close your eyes.

For beginners

Sit on a cushion if you cannot sit straight comfortably.

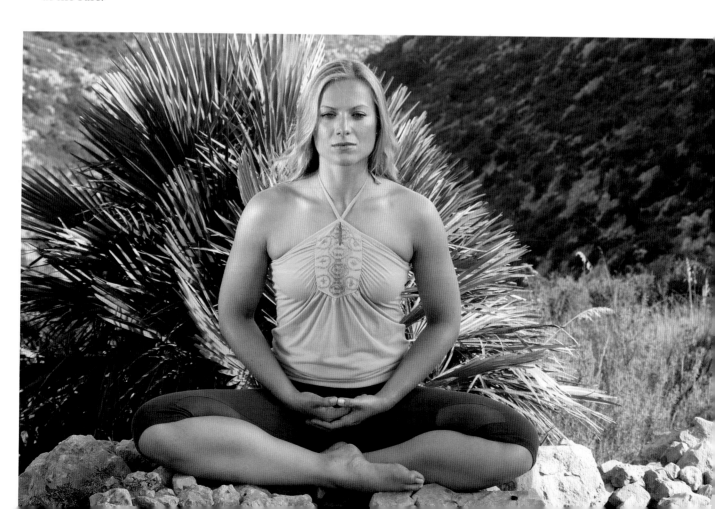

Vìrasana Hero Pose

In this position – like Vajrasana (opposite) – the spine is held straight upright and stretched; however, it does also require a certain degree of flexibility in the hips. The body remains centred and calm, making this asana suitable for switching off for a short time, allowing you to gather your thoughts, concentrate or meditate.

Alignment

- Kneel down with your feet just over hip-width apart. Use a hand to push your calves gently back and out (see detailed view (a)); allow enough space to be able to sit between your feet (see detailed view (b)). The tops of your feet should be flat on the floor and your feet should be close to your hips.

- Allow your sit bones and hips to sink to the floor and keep your knees together.

- Straighten your spine and pull up through the crown of your head. Keep your back straight, particularly at the base.

- Rest your hands in your lap or on your thighs. Look gently down or close your eyes.

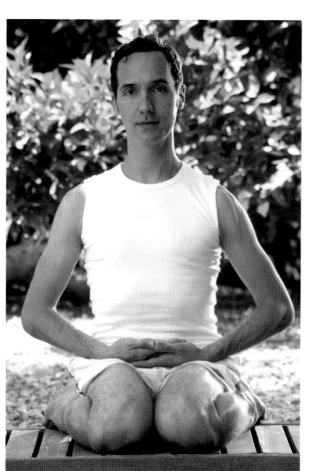

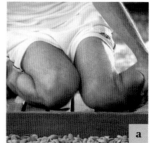 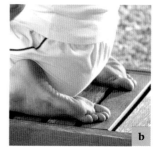

Detailed views

For beginners ▼

a. Sit on a block if you find it uncomfortable sitting on the floor.

b. And/or use a belt to keep your knees together.

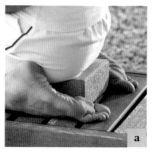 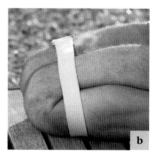

vajrasana Thunderbolt Pose

Thunderbolt Pose is an alternative to Sukhasana (see p.202) or Siddhasana/Muktasana (see p.203). However, it does require an element of flexibility in the knees. The main benefit of this position is that it keeps the spine straight and stretched. The body is centred and calmed, making this asana ideal for switching off for a short time, allowing you to gather your thoughts, concentrate or meditate.

Alignment

- Kneel down, resting the tops of your feet on the floor and with your bottom on your heels.

- Straighten your spine and pull up through the crown of your head. Keep your back straight, particularly at the base.

- Rest your hands on your thighs, and look into the distance or close your eyes.

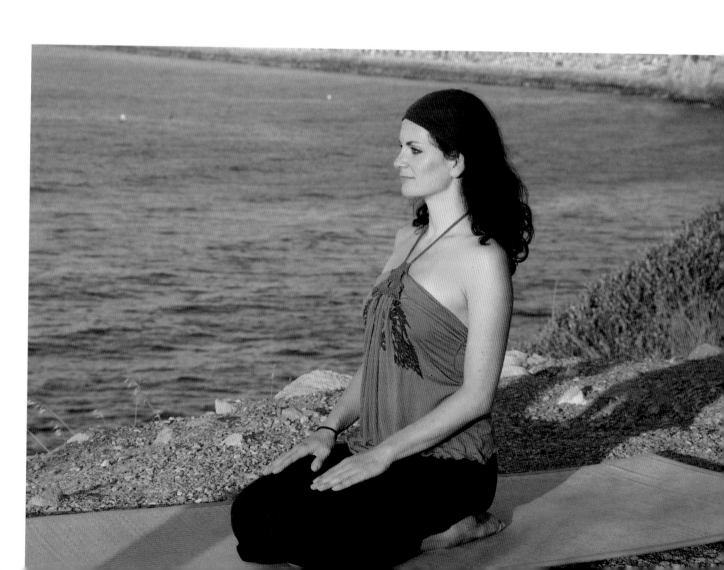

padmasana Lotus
ardha padmasana Half Lotus
baddha padmasana Bound Lotus

The Lotus is the classic meditation position, but does require rather a lot of practice and flexibility in the hips, knees and ankles. Once you have mastered the pose, it can be very relaxing, as the body becomes centred, calm and stable. The position of the legs keeps the spine straight almost by itself, allowing it to relax.

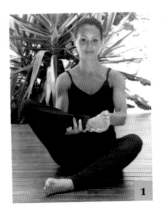
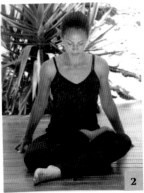
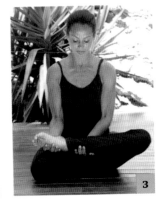
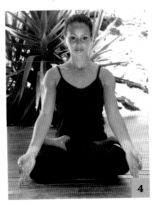

Ardha Padmasana

Padmasana

Step-by-step alignment

1. Take one arm under your calf, grab hold of your foot and lift it up. Open up your hips by turning the thigh and knee of your upper leg gently outwards.

2. Lay your foot with the sole facing upwards in the opposite groin (not on the thigh muscle). Place your heel as close as possible to your navel. This position is called Ardha Padmasana: the Half Lotus.

3. Take hold of your other leg under the calf and grab hold of your foot. Turn your knee gently outwards.

4. Lay this foot with the sole facing upwards in the other groin. Place your heel as close as possible to your navel. Allow your sit bones, hips and knees to sink to the floor. Keep your spine straight and stretch up through the crown of your head. Keep your back straight, particularly at the base. Lay the backs of your hands against your knees and position your hands in Jnana mudra (see p.39).

5. Alternatively, cross your arms behind your back, bring your hands round to the front and take hold of your toes. This is Baddha Padmasana: the Bound Lotus.

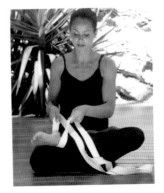

◄ For beginners

Practise the Half Lotus (Step 2) until you can sit comfortably in this position for some time. Then, using a belt, place the ankle of the other leg in the bend of your knee until you can put your foot in your groin.

Baddha Padmasana ►

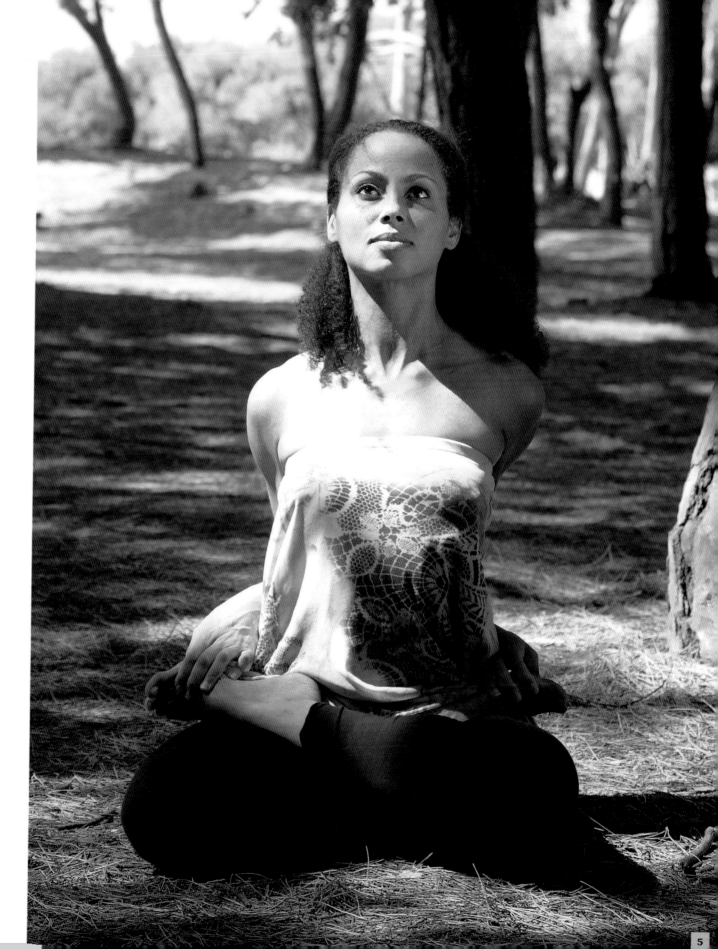

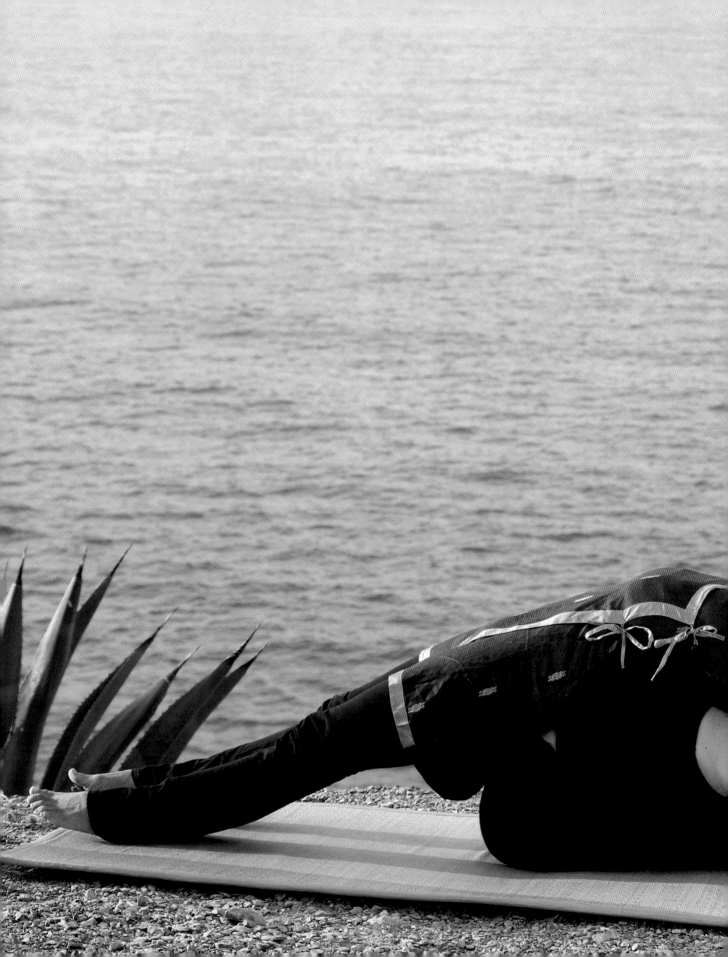

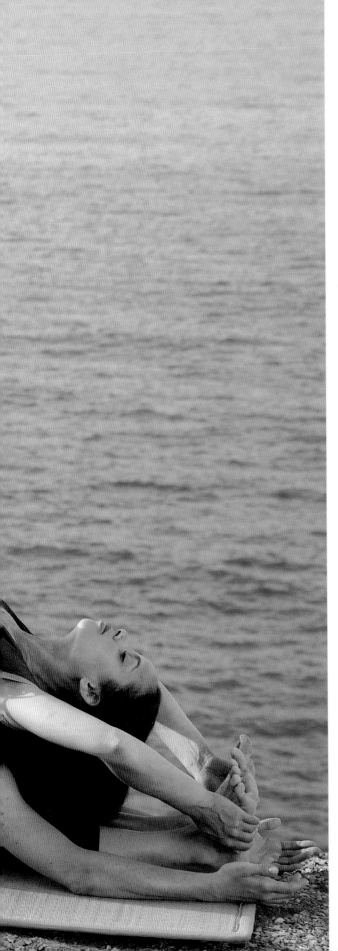

Relaxing postures

As their name implies, these postures are first and foremost aimed at relaxation. The main purpose is to relax the spine, which is responsible for bearing the body's weight in the course of daily life as well as during yoga practice.

Physiologically, relaxation postures restore balance after intense asana practice. They also provide deep relaxation of the whole body and have a very restorative effect. In this state of relaxation, the body feels heavy but floppy at the same time, and as you practise the asanas, the body sinks deep into the floor.

On an emotional level, relaxation positions help you to let go. The mind releases the body and thoughts, and becomes light and unencumbered. So the postures can also provide 'islands of peace' in the stormy seas of daily life and can be practised at any time. These postures make it possible for you to gather your thoughts and relax, not just in the context of asana practice, but whenever you need to do so.

balasana   Child's Pose

Child's Pose, also called Folded Leaf Pose, is frequently adopted while practising asanas to provide brief relaxation. It is also useful for gathering your thoughts for a short time and looking deeper into your 'inner self'. It addition, it is a good neutralizing position after gentle backbends. The spine, including the cervical vertebrae, is stretched and relaxed.

Alignment

- Assume Vajrasana (see p.205) and bend your upper body forwards. Lay your forehead on the floor and relax your arms by the sides of your body.

- Push your tailbone down and feel the length and space of your whole spine.

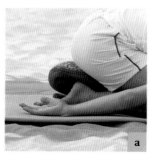

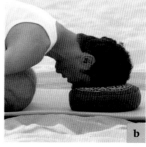

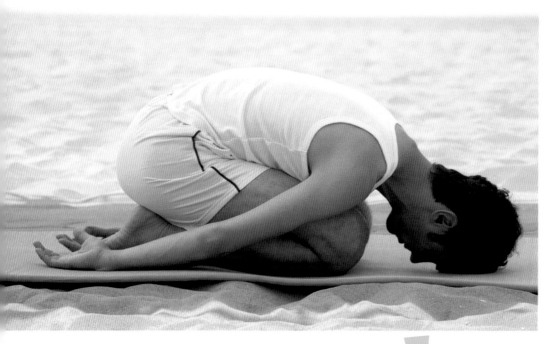

In Balasana you feel secure because the pose reflects the embryo position.

For beginners

a. If your bottom does not touch your heels, place a cushion between them.

b. If you cannot lay your forehead comfortably on the floor, use a cushion.

apanāsana   Knees to Chest Pose

In this position the whole spine, especially the lower back, is stretched and relaxed, making it an ideal neutralizing position to assume after backbends. It is also a good posture to assume at any time of day, particularly after standing or sitting for a long time.

Alignment

- Lie with your back flat on the floor, bend your legs and use both arms to pull your knees towards your body.

- Raise your upper body from the floor and take your nose to your knees. Keep your middle and lower back in contact with the floor. Rock backwards and forwards, giving your back a gentle massage.

- Lay your hands on your knees, and as you inhale, push your knees away from your body. As you exhale, pull them back to the body.

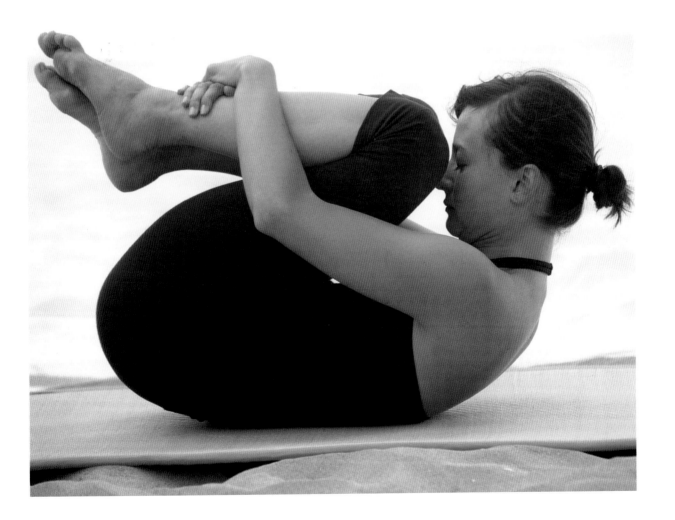

Happy Baby Pose

Happy Baby Pose is one of the few asanas that do not have a Sanskrit name. The whole spine, particularly the lower back, is stretched and relaxed. This makes it an ideal neutralizing position after forward and backward bends. Many people also find that opening the hips wide in this asana makes it even more relaxing.

Alignment

- Lie flat on your back, and as you inhale, bend your knees.

- Take hold of your toes, and as you exhale, pull your knees down towards the floor. Keep your whole back on the floor.

- Rock from side to side like a happy baby, giving your back a gentle massage.

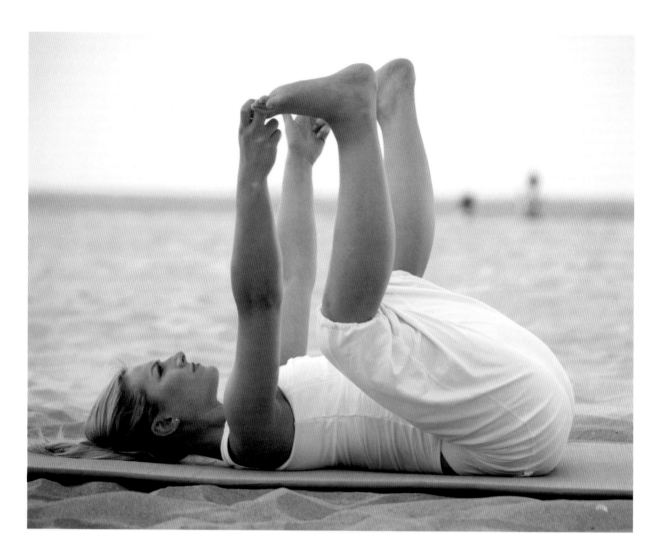

jathara parivartanasana **Reclined Twist**

Although the spine is not straight but twisted in this position, this is still a relaxation posture and is very pleasant after intense asana practice. It is particularly beneficial for neutralizing the spine after forward and backward bends.

Alignment

- Lie flat on your back. Roll onto one hip and bend the upper leg. As you exhale, use the hand on the other side of your body to guide your upper leg over your lower leg down to the floor. Keep your hips straight and the muscles in your lower leg tense.

- Place your hand on your knee and push it gently down to the floor.

- Stretch your other arm out to the side and look towards your fingertips. Keep both shoulders on the floor.

For beginners ▼

Place a cushion under your knee if you cannot get it to the floor.

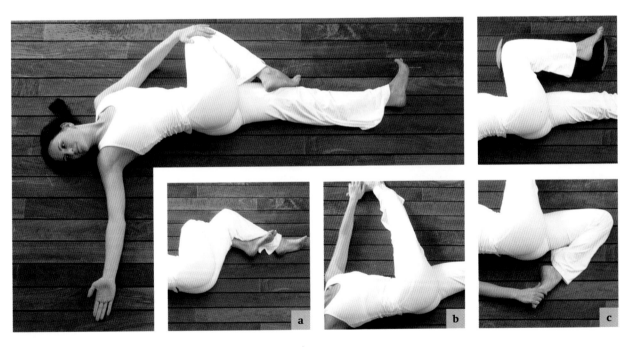

For advanced students ▲

a. Cross your legs for a pleasant additional stretch in the hips.

b. Take hold of your toes and stretch your upper leg to get an intense stretch in the rear thigh muscle.

c. As well as holding onto your toes, you can also bend your lower leg and pull it gently in the direction of your bottom, to achieve a stretch in the front thigh muscle of the bent leg.

supta baddha konasana Reclining Bound Angle Pose

This posture allows the spine to relax in a neutral position and release the weight of the whole body to the floor. At the same time, the position of the legs opens the hips and relaxes the buttocks. This is a beneficial posture during menstruation and for relieving abdominal discomfort.

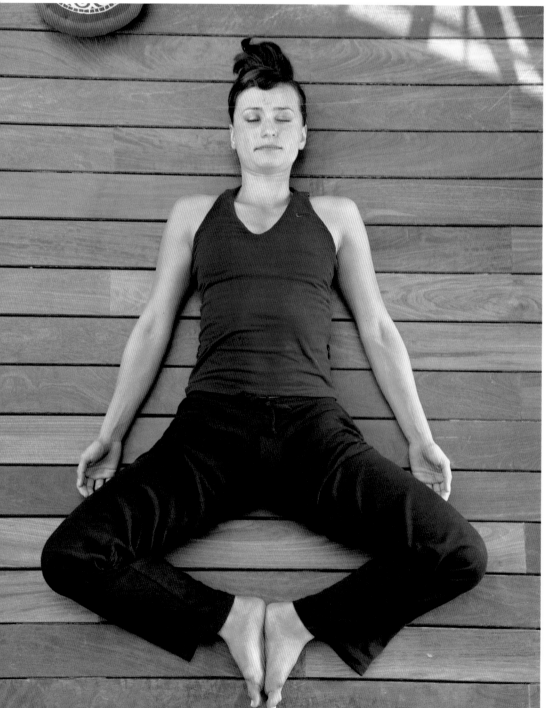

Alignment

- Lie flat on your back, bend your legs and place the soles of your feet together.

- Allow your knees to fall out to the sides and sink to the floor, and relax your arms alongside your body. Close your eyes.

For beginners ▼

If you cannot lie comfortably on the floor, support yourself on your forearms. Place cushions under your knees if you are not able to sink them right down to the floor.

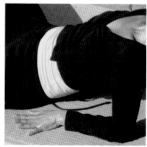

ꣵavaꣵana   Corpse Pose

Corpse Pose symbolises letting go of the body and mind, so it is the most effective relaxation position of all. The whole body is relaxed and motionless, and the pelvis and shoulders in particular release all their tension within. The inner mental relaxation – the letting go of all thought while remaining alert – acts like a fountain of youth on the body and spirit.

Alignment

- Lie flat on your back. Allow your legs and feet to fall gently apart.

- Let your arms relax alongside your body with your palms facing upwards and close your eyes. Relax your face and let yourself sink deep into the floor. Enjoy the position.

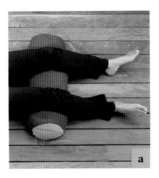
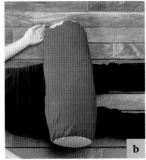

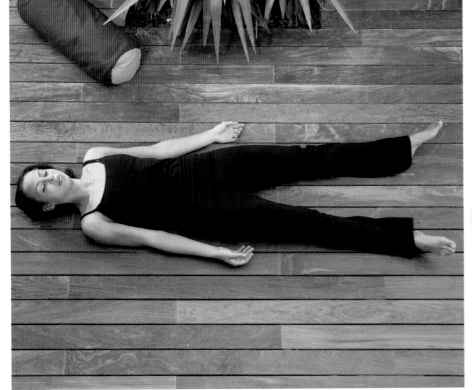

Variations ▲

a. Place a cushion under the backs of your knees to relax your lower back.

b. Lay a cushion on top of your hips to help you sink deeper into the floor.

Something that sounds so easy – namely letting everything go and staying conscious and alert without falling asleep or thinking – requires a certain amount of practice. If thoughts do start coming into your head, do not let them influence you: simply allow them to drift over you and do not pursue them.

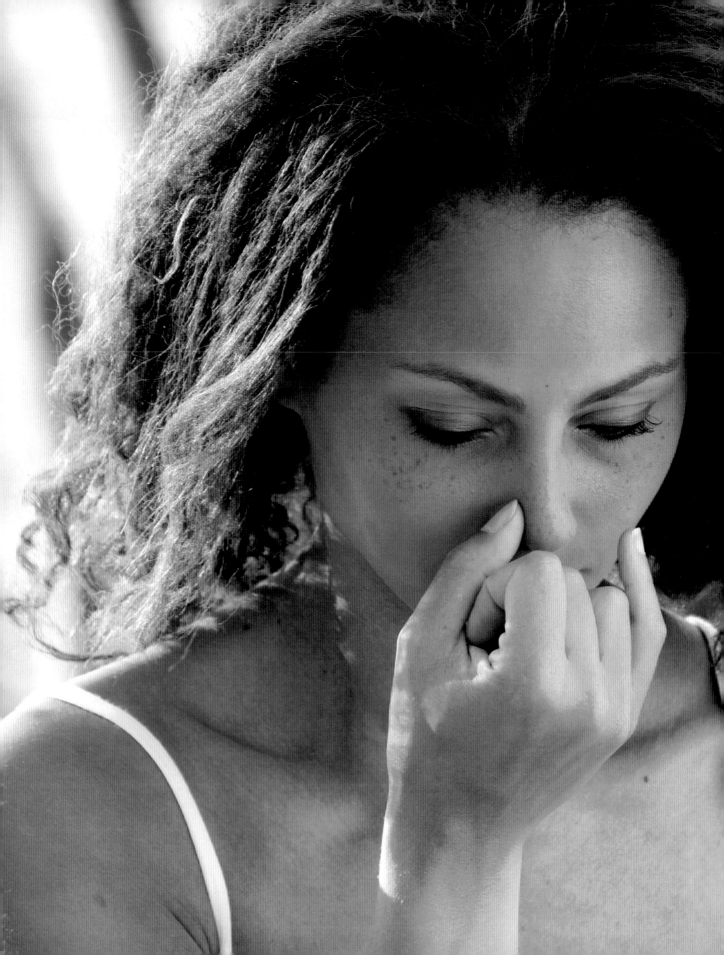

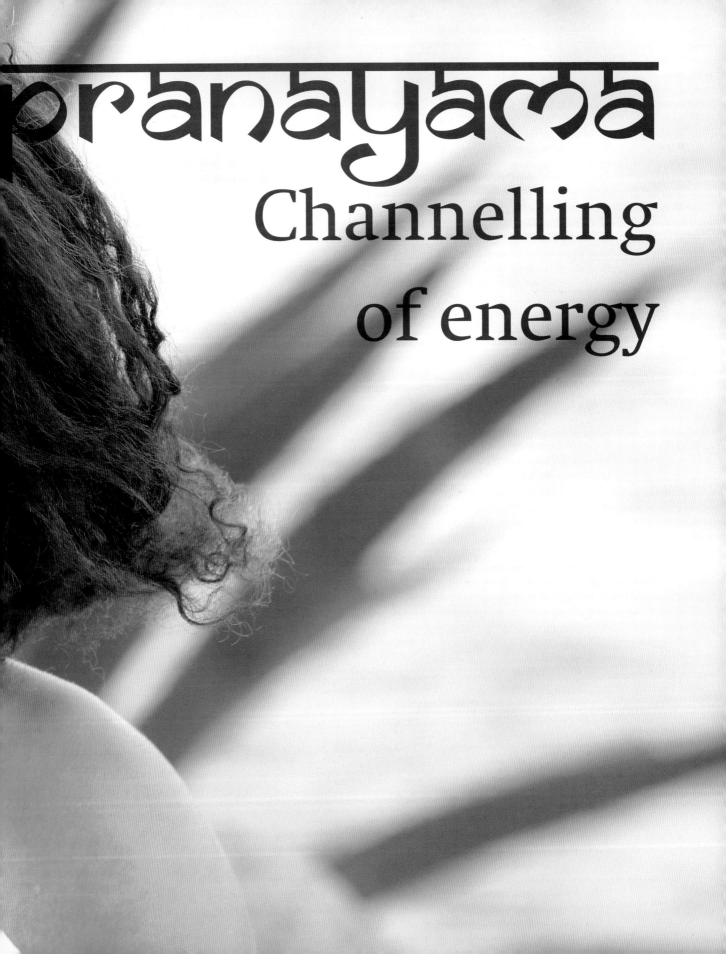

pranayama

Channelling
of energy

The nature and goal of pranayama

Breath: The mirror of the body and mind

In our daily lives, our breathing frequently reflects our state of mind. Each thought and feeling expresses itself in the form of relaxation or tension, peace or worry, receptiveness or fear, and triggers a biochemical reaction in the body. In normal speech too, there are many expressions that relate to the relationship between the body, mind and breathing: you catch your breath, something takes your breath away, you wait with bated breath, you take a breather, or you come up for air – are just a few examples. If you are relaxed, your breathing is regular, deep and calm. However, if you are in inner turmoil, for whatever reason, your breathing becomes shallow, rapid and irregular.

Pranayama: Channelling of energy

The Sanskrit word *pranayama* has a variety of meanings: *pra* means 'movement'; *na* means 'continuous' or 'persistent'; *prana* means 'energy'; *yama* means 'control' or 'guidance'; and *ayama* means 'spreading' or 'expansion'. So the best translation is either 'energy channelling' or 'energy expansion'. Pranayama is achieved through the breath.

Pranayama brings about a calm mind

In the same way as the mind affects the breath, the breath influences the mind. This is the exact function of pranayama, which is the fourth stage of Patanjali's Eight-Limb Path, and a central part of yoga practice in Hatha Yoga (see pp.32–9). Practised over thousands of years, these techniques are consciously controlled breathing exercises that bring about beneficial changes in the body and mind. They help to achieve mental and physical calm and to get rid of or overcome obstructions in the energetic body. Conscious changes to the normally unconscious pattern of breathing not only facilitate a union between the mind, body and breath, but also create vital energy in the body and mind (see box, above right).

Conscious breathing

There is hardly anything that is more automatic and less controlled than natural breathing, and barely anything to which we pay as little attention as this vital activity. Natural breathing is often shallow and irregular and punctuated with unconscious pauses, which reflect an absent-minded, unfocused or stressed mind. And it is not easy to observe your breathing without changing your natural breathing pattern. The breaths usually deepen automatically as soon as you start concentrating and focusing on them. But conscious breathing – the observation of the natural breath without changing it – is the preliminary stage for any breathing exercise, in order to be able to understand one's own mental and physical state and experience the effects of a subsequent breathing exercise.

> ## Prana – life force
>
> *In yoga, prana means 'vital energy' or 'life force'. The aim is to unite the inner, which is always present, with the outer, which is nourished with food, intellectual stimuli, movement and breathing. The goal of pranayama therefore is to enrich the body with vital energy and 'recharge its batteries'.*
>
> *To derive the greatest possible benefit from this energy, it must be able to circulate around the body unimpeded. If you pursue a healthy lifestyle and can relax without too many worries, the vital energy circulates freely. However, tensions and blockages that arise in the body as a result of too much stress and strain prevent the life force from flowing freely. This results in prana not being kept in the body where it can be circulated, but draining away with no effect. Prana circulates in the nadis, the energy channels within the body (see p.35). Practising yoga asanas and pranayama helps to clear these channels, allowing the energy to remain in the body and flow freely.*

The four phases of breathing

Natural and controlled breathing have four phases:
- Inhalation (Sanskrit *puraka*)
- Pause after inhalation (Sanskrit *antara kumbhaka*)
- Exhalation (Sanskrit *rechaka*)
- Pause after exhalation (Sanskrit *bahya kumbhaka*)

Pauses between breaths, also called breath retention (or *kumbhaka* in Sanskirt), are generally very short, but in breathing exercises can be consciously lengthened.

Putting pranayama into practice

Performing breathing exercises after practising asanas is good preparation for meditation, as pranayama is also perceived as a bridge between the body and the mind. Some of the techniques on the following pages can also be carried out before you begin your yoga asanas, while others are perfect for combining with asana practice (see box below). You will find suggestions with the relevant breathing exercises.

Caution recommended

If you are not yet familiar with the breathing exercises, you should first practise with a qualified yoga teacher. Once you have practised a little, you will be able to perform the techniques on your own. But you should always proceed with caution: take pranayama exercises slowly and step by step, because in some circumstances incorrect breathing can result in feelings of dizziness.

Ujjayi – breathing during asana practice

'Ujjayi' means 'the victorious breath' in Sanskrit, and this protracted breathing technique produces even, deep and regulated in- and out-breaths through the nose, generally without consciously holding the breath. It is produced by narrowing the larynx and glottis – similar to whispering, but with a closed mouth – so that a gentle noise, like the sound of the sea, is heard. This breathing is generally used during asana practice and is co-ordinated with movement. Each inhalation and exhalation is of equal length and starts and finishes the movement.

Meditation in movement: with a certain amount of practice, you can put yourself into a virtually meditative state by combining Ujjayi breathing and asana practice. This helps to maintain the

concentration and mental focus. Breathing brings attentiveness and consciousness to the moment and prevents your mind from wandering too easily.

With the help of Ujjayi breathing, advanced students can consciously direct the breath into specific parts of the body – for instance, 'breathing into the hip' – to dissolve energy blockages in specific areas, as well as to perceive boundaries. It is therefore also called an inner teacher, because it prompts you to take breaks and withdraw whenever calm and regular breathing is no longer possible: this is always indicative of physical barriers that you will encounter as you practise, which must be respected. With a little practice and patience you will find you can perform increasingly complex asanas.

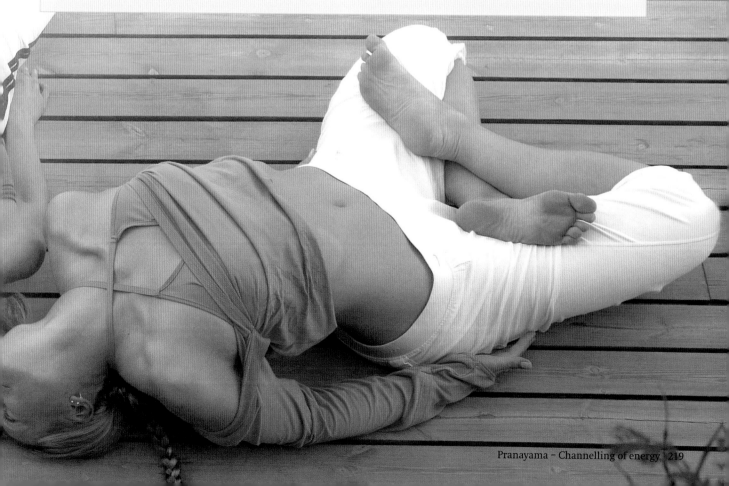

The most important pranayama exercises

Three-part yogic breathing: stomach-chest-shoulders

This classic yoga exercise is particularly suitable for initiating conscious breathing at the start of an asana session. As you inhale and exhale, the path of the breath is followed on its course through the body, enabling the individual airways to be felt and consciously filled (see below for instructions).

Instructions for three-part yogic breathing

This breathing exercise can be practised while standing, sitting or lying down.

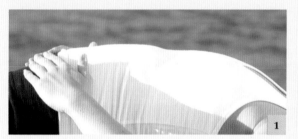

Lay your hands on your stomach and breathe consciously through your nose into your stomach, so that you can feel it expanding in all directions.

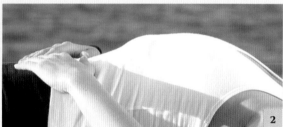

Release the breath from your stomach back through your nose, pulling your navel gently in and up.

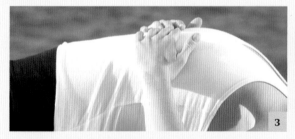

Lay your hands on your ribcage and breathe consciously through your nose into your chest, so that your chest expands in all directions.

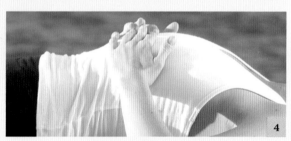

Expel the breath back through your nose and lower your ribcage.

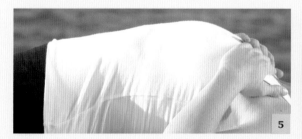

Lay your hands on your collarbones and breathe consciously through your nose into your shoulder area, so that it expands in all directions.

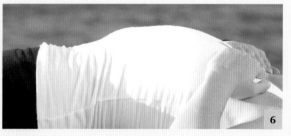

Expel the breath back out of your shoulder area through your nose and lower your collarbones.

Observe how the breath enters and is expelled from the individual parts of the body. With a little practice you will be able to direct one third of a single breath to the stomach, one third to the chest and one third to the shoulders, enabling you to feel all three areas at the same time.

Instructions for Nadi Shodhana

- *Breathe slowly in and out through both nostrils several times.*

- *Ensure that your head remains level and take one hand to your nose. Right-handers should use their right hand, and left-handers their left.*

- *Choose one of the following two hand positions to close the right and left nostrils in turn: fold down your index and middle fingers and regulate your in-breaths by closing off the nostril either underneath (see images, right) or directly below the bridge of your nose (see images, below).*

- *Close off your right nostril and inhale through your left nostril. Close off your left nostril and exhale through your right nostril. Inhale through your right nostril, close off your right nostril and exhale through your left nostril.*

- *Repeat this cycle with even inhalations and exhalations. If you like, slowly increase the length of your breaths. Finish the exercise by exhaling from your left nostril.*

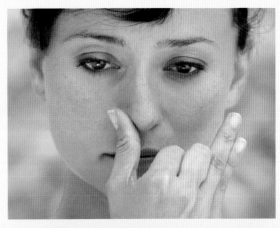

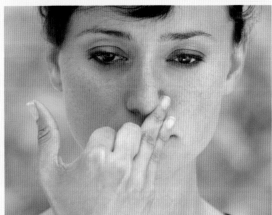

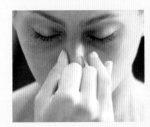
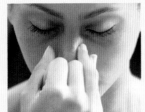

Nadi Shodhana pranayama – Alternate Nostril Breathing

The literal translation of this breathing technique is 'cleansing of the nadis', the energy channels (see p.35). It is also called alternate nostril breathing, because you inhale and exhale through alternate nostrils, with both sides of the body working in harmony. In Hatha Yoga, the sun's energy is associated with the right nostril; the male side is associated with qualities such as energy, warmth, intellect and activity (see p.32). The moon's energy is female, and the left nostril is the channel for its associated qualities of coolness, passivity, emotions and intuition. Alternate nostril breathing aims to balance and harmonize the two forms of energy (see box above for instructions).

This breathing technique is usually performed after asana practice in preparation for meditation. However, alternate nostril breathing can be performed any time to bring about a sense of calmness and peace.

Samavritti pranayama – Regular Breathing

With regular breathing, all the phases of breathing (the inhalation, the pause after inhalation, the exhalation and the pause after exhalation) are the same length and of the same intensity. Beginners can start with three or four counts per breathing phase, and more advanced students can increase to eight counts. This balancing breathing exercise can be carried out at any time with or without breath retention.

Visamavritti pranayama – Irregular Breathing

With irregular breathing, either the inhalation or exhalation is accentuated and carried out for longer, for example, inhalation for three counts and exhalation for six counts. The number of counts can slowly be increased. If the inhalation is accentuated, the exercise has an invigorating effect; if the exhalation is accentuated, the effect is calming. This breathing technique can be carried out at any time.

Sitali and sitkari – breath-cooling exercise

This breathing exercise can be practised with the tongue curled and protruding slightly from the mouth (sitali) or flat and pressed back against the roof of the mouth (sitkari), depending upon personal preference (and ability). Inhale slowly either through the opening in the tongue or between the teeth; exhale equally slowly through both nostrils. This exercise cools the body, and has a revitalizing and refreshing effect.

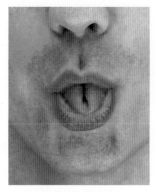 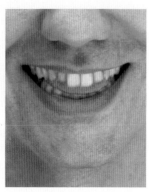

Sitali – cooling breath with curled tongue   *Sitkari – cooling breath with tongue pressed back*

Surya Bedhana – sun breath

In the sun breath, you inhale through your right nostril and exhale through your left (see box, p.221). Breathing is regular, in other words the inhalation and exhalation are of equal length. This exercise has an energizing, energy-burning and warming effect, and can be practised whenever you feel tired or cold inside.

Chandra Bedhana – moon breath

In the moon breath, you inhale through your left nostril and exhale through your right (see box, p.221). Breathing is regular, in other words the inhalation and exhalation are of equal length. This exercise has a calming and cooling effect and can be practised whenever you feel nervous, uneasy or hot inside.

Viloma pranayama – unnatural breath

In Viloma pranayama (literally, 'breathing against the natural order of things'), the inhalation or exhalation is punctuated by holding your breath for an equal length of time; e.g. inhale for two counts, hold your breath for two counts, then continue inhaling for two counts, hold your breath to a count of two, finally continuing to inhale for two counts, before letting out your breath in one full exhalation. Or vice versa. If the inhalation is interrupted, the effect of the exercise is energizing; if the exhalation is interrupted, the effect is calming and relaxing. This breathing exercise is predominantly for more advanced students, since breath retention requires a lot of practice.

Bastrika – bellows breath

Bastrika means 'bellows' in Sanskrit, and this breathing exercise actually creates a sound similar to that produced by bellows: as you breathe in and out, the air is powerfully sucked in and then expelled (this is one cycle). The number of cycles should be increased slowly and carefully, if necessary incorporating pauses. Bellows breathing strengthens and stimulates the digestive organs and stomach muscles, and cleanses the sinuses.

Kapalabhati – cleaning breath

Kapalabhati is one of the cleansing rituals (see Shat Karma Kriya p.38), but is also a gentler version of bastrika. It is only the exhalation that requires the air to be expelled explosively by powerful contractions of the abdominal wall, similar to blowing your nose. Once the abdominal wall is released again, the inhalation happens normally and naturally. The exercise and effects are the same as bastrika.

Bastrika and kapalabhati generate heat and have an energizing and cleansing effect. However, the forced breathing is strenuous and should be practised with caution, even by advanced students. If you suffer from high blood pressure or experience discomfort in the stomach area you should not practise these exercises.

The full Uddiyana bandha

In this exercise, Uddiyana bandha is practised and strengthened using an intensive breathing technique. The full Uddiyana bandha invigorates the whole abdominal area and organs, strengthens the digestive system and stimulates detoxification of the digestive organs (see box below for step-by-step instructions). To learn how to perform this exercise correctly you must seek the advice of a teacher. The full Uddiyana bandha can be practised at any time – but only on an empty stomach, as the exercise can otherwise be rather unpleasant. The ideal time is in the morning, immediately after getting up.

Instructions for the full Uddiyana bandha

- *Stand with your legs hip-width apart and your knees slightly bent. Inhale deeply through your nose, and pull your pelvic floor up (Mula bandha, see p.52).*

- *As you exhale, bend forward and place your hands on your thighs, keeping your arms straight. Exhale through your mouth and stick your tongue out.*

- *Lock your throat (Jalandhara bandha, see p.53) and expand your chest, as if inhaling, but without allowing air to flow in through your throat. This creates a vacuum in your chest and your stomach will be sucked in deep under the ribs. The full Uddiyana bandha happens automatically and there is no need to contract the muscles.*

- *At this point, hold your breath for a moment and try to pull your navel further in and up.*

- *Release Uddiyana bandha first, then Jalandhara bandha and finally Mula bandha.*

- *Inhale deeply through your nose and straighten up again. Repeat the exercise several times.*

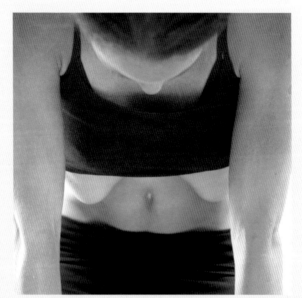

Full Uddiyana bandha from the front

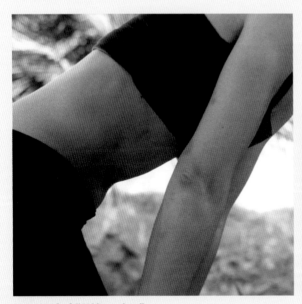

Preparing for full Uddiyana bandha

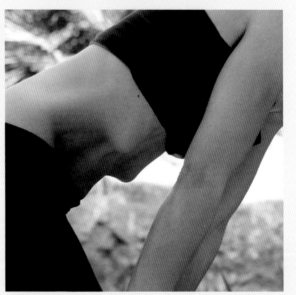

A vacuum in the abdominal area causes full Uddiyana bandha to occur automatically as you hold your breath

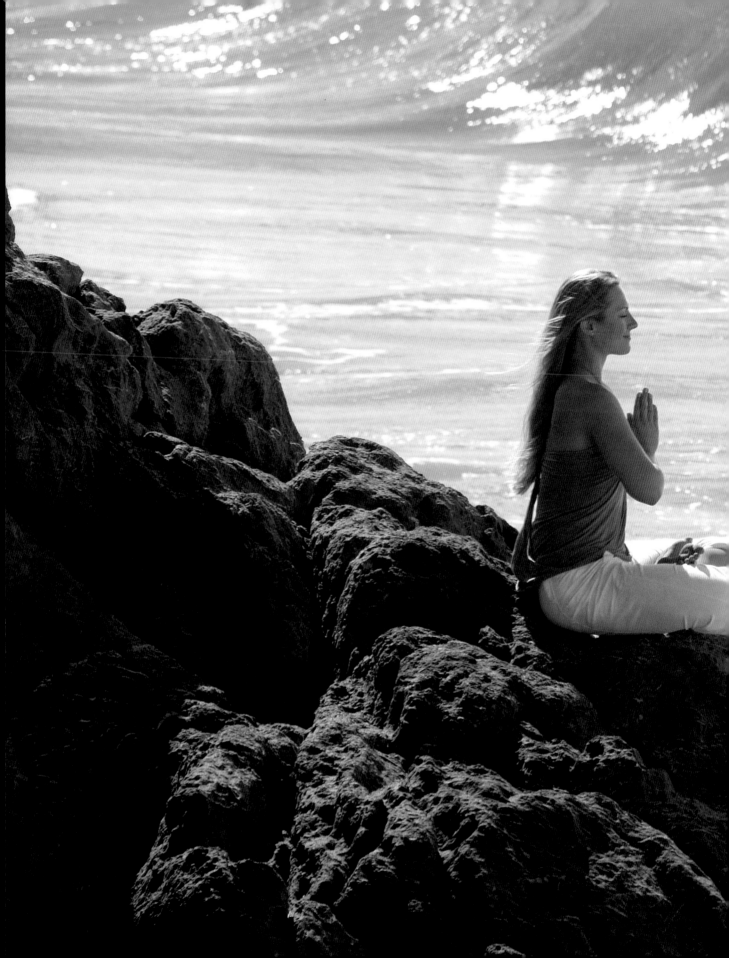

dhyana
Meditation

The nature and goal of meditation

Meditation – a tried-and-tested method

For more than 2,000 years, meditation has been practised in numerous countries and by a wide range of cultures as an effective means of allowing people to look into their innermost selves. Today, it is often used in the West, predominantly to calm the mind and find inner peace and composure. This means that meditation has something to offer those looking for spirituality as well as those with a more pragmatic approach who may have no interest in spiritual matters.

However, the benefits of meditation extend far beyond this: meditation also involves focusing on a chosen object for the duration of a session. This may be yourself, another person, an object, a situation, a word, a feeling, or just your own body or breath. Concentrating exclusively on the object and being aware of all changes during this observation without reacting to them: this is the essence of any meditation, the aim being to learn something about yourself or others, and life in general.

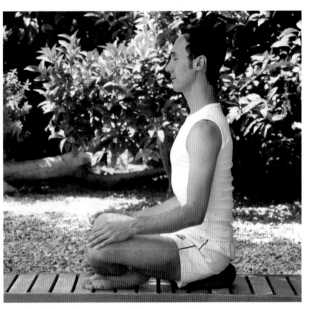

A comfortable meditation pose: Sukhasana, Easy Pose

Finding concentration

The mind has a tendency to be restless, flitting from one thought to the next. Most thoughts go through our minds thousands of times in a similar form without developing further or going any deeper. So it does no harm to deviate from those well-worn paths of thought and your own thought patterns, to experience yourself from a different perspective, to listen to your inner self, and to seek out your own fundamental nature. The idea of simply sitting there and not doing anything may at first seem a little strange and perhaps even difficult. However, with a little practice you will find that it becomes easier to allow yourself a small oasis of calm where you can focus the mind and find concentration.

The goal: enlightenment

Meditation (*dhyana*) is the seventh stage of Patanjali's Eight-Limb Path (see p.31). The goal of meditation is to reach samadhi, the eighth stage – realization or enlightenment. In Hatha Yoga (see pp.32–9), it is also an important part of yoga practice on the path to enlightenment. Realization comes about and is experienced in an extremely personal way that can only be put into words in a very general sense. For example, some people speak of barriers being removed, while

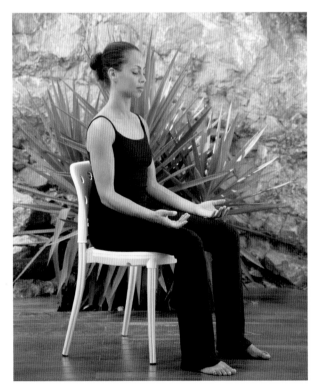

A simple meditation pose: Egyptian Posture

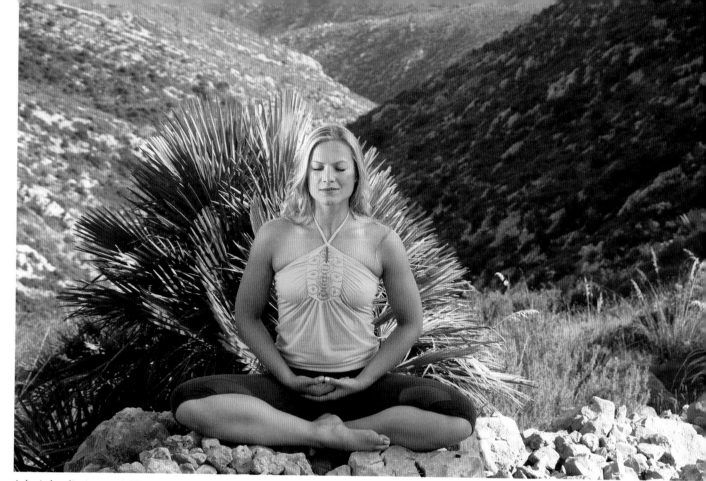

A classical meditation pose: Siddhasana, Perfect Pose

others say that it is as if they become fused with the object of their meditation. Descriptions of deep-reaching meditations try to convey the changed energy experience whereby the person breathing and the breath becoming breathing itself. In classical yoga literature, there are numerous other descriptions of meditation experiences, in which the end result is described as an integrated state of existence-consciousness-bliss (*sat-chit-ananda*).

The positive effects of meditation

The mind is often compared to an ocean whose surface is moved by permanent waves of thoughts. If the thoughts come to rest, the ocean becomes calm and clear, until the bottom is visible once more. Things can be seen as they really are, without distortion or cloudiness. This is exactly what meditation can achieve. Meditation produces all kinds of effects, and with some practice, some or all of the beneficial results mentioned here can be experienced.

Meditation:
- *strengthens the body and recharges the batteries;*
- *leads to peace and tranquillity, equilibrium and balance;*
- *enhances the powers of concentration and capability;*
- *improves general physical, mental and spiritual well-being;*
- *delves deep into the depths of one's own personality to discover the true self;*
- *raises self-awareness and self-confidence, and allows you to see your own strengths so as to make better use of them. In the same way, weaknesses are better understood and accepted;*
- *helps you to understand your needs better, nurturing the concept of being 'good to yourself';*
- *provides deep realization of the properties and qualities of universal existence and consciousness.*

Meditation: Inner retreat

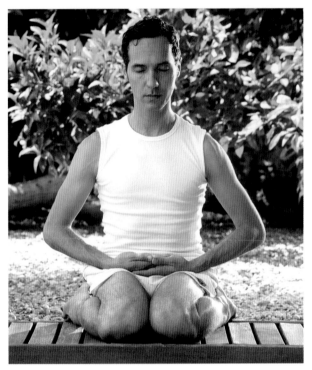

Only recommended if you do not suffer from knee problems: the meditation pose Virasana, Hero Pose

Access to deeper levels of consciousness

Meditation is first and foremost, but by no means only, for relaxation. It leads to a form of inner retreat or introspection that opens up a new path to deeper understanding of oneself, others or a favourite object. Meditation enables you to probe into inner areas to which access is usually denied in a normal state of mind. During meditation, previously unknown or unsensed emotions and feelings can be experienced and deciphered – almost like a message from the subconscious.

If during meditation we concentrate on our own pattern of reactions and habits, we will recognize their origins. This will bring us deeper knowledge of our past.
(Yoga Sutra 3.18.)

Objects of meditation

The object of meditation can be anything at all. However, it is best to select an object that is connected to you, or to a relevant situation – depending upon what you need to understand at the time. These can be feelings, behavioural traits, situations, other people, objects, or simply your own breath, body, or individual parts of your body – or even just a single word. Practising meditation actually involves doing nothing more than observing, but not reacting to, the impulses sent out by the body, mind and spirit. By observing these impulses, the realization grows that they are influenced by many things – namely experiences, ideas, wishes and fears. What happens initially is that all of these influences divert your thoughts and feelings into well-worn patterns; however, if you observe the impulses for long enough and watch them in their never-ending movements, you will be able to experience individual moments relating to the particular object of meditation among the general non-discriminate melee. At this stage, thought and feeling can be said to cross the barriers of 'well-trodden paths' and find new paths; the object is perceived in a different light and the observer – the self – gains new insights.

If an elephant is the object of meditation, the strength of the elephant can arise in oneself.
(Yoga Sutra 2.24.)

Key principles of meditation

The key principles for concentrating on a particular object can be summarized as follows: release, observe, evaluate nothing. This sums up the three most important aspects of meditation.

Release

In meditation you need to let go; this means on the one hand, not forcing anything – no thought, feeling, perception – but, equally, not suppressing anything, not even the faintest inner emotion. Letting go means giving up every desire and every intent, and therefore, in the positive sense, your control over all internal and external events, but particularly the desire to reach immediate enlightenment. As you allow your feelings, thoughts, emotions and sensations to well up, new inner messages will open up to you during your meditation.

Observation

The second important aspect of any meditation is to observe, but not to react to, these unbidden thoughts and feelings, memories or anything else. Not reacting means not responding to what you have observed, either by an uncontrolled movement (i.e. with the body) or with a thought (i.e. with the mind), because every response triggers new feelings and thoughts, setting a never-ending chain reaction in motion. Instead, the idea is to allow everything that comes to mind in the way of inner pictures and sensations to pass by like clouds in the sky – as if you are completely remote from it all.

Not evaluating anything

Whatever inner pictures and messages might come to the surface and enter the consciousness during the course of a meditation, they all have a right to do so. Because as you probe deeper into an object, word, living entity or quality, or come to recognize it in all of its facets, there is nothing that is 'right' or 'wrong'. This is why the third key principle of every meditation is not evaluating anything as being good or bad, horrible or nice, pleasant or painful and commenting on it internally, but seeing all feelings and all thoughts as equal, and – as the mind is constantly in motion – also letting them go again.

A comfortable meditation pose for many people: Vajrasana, Thunderbolt Pose

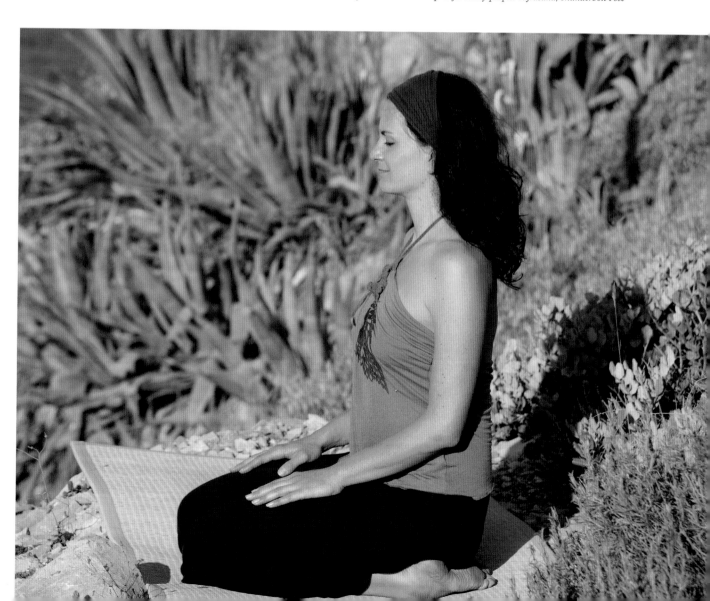

Different kinds of meditation

Meditation with and without concrete focus

There are basically two kinds of meditation: concrete meditation (*saguna*), in which a specific characteristic serves as a focus for the concentration and attention; and abstract meditation (*nirguna*), which has no specific characteristic and is formless. Each kind does not necessarily preclude the other. On the contrary, it is highly possible to float across from a concrete meditation into a non-concrete, semi-abstract form of meditation.

Breath meditation

Concentration on breathing is often regarded as the gateway to meditation. After a while breathing becomes more regular and calm – almost automatically. This breathing pattern also affects the mind, which becomes calmer and peaceful, and no longer forms a barrier against advancing into deeper levels of awareness.

Body meditation

Concentrating on the whole body or specific parts of the body, such as the space between the eyebrows ('the third eye') or the heart area, is a classic meditation exercise. It enables parts of the body to be explored and experienced, and stress or blockages in energy to be exposed and partially or completely cleansed. These may be purely physical, or they may be emotional stress too, which can also cause physical tensions.

Mudra meditation

Mudra means 'seal' and refers to the positions of the hands, fingers, eyes or tongue (see p.39). Mudras encourage concentration on the energy flow through the body and the conscious awareness of this energy.

Mantra meditation

A mantra (from the Sanskrit *man* for 'mind' and *tra* for 'tool') can be a syllable, word or sentence. Mantras can be used in meditation – like a tool. Each mantra contains a kind of energy, rather like a frequency that you tune into on the radio to receive a station. Depending on the 'frequency' of a mantra, various energies can be released in the meditation and effects generated – for example, energy, weightlessness or an opening of the heart. Mantras are usually recited or chanted in constant repetition. A classic mantra that encourages the heart to open and reveal sensations such as love and empathy, as well as being able to dissolve emotional blockages is:

OM *mane peme hung*
('Hail to the jewel in the lotus')

Visualization

By concentrating on a picture or visual concept, visualizing meditation offers numerous ways to develop and absorb energies from that visual image and to find new strength. A picture or concept – for example, the picture of a tiger or even an abstract concept such as 'light' – enables the relevant information, qualities and attributes to be internalized and experienced piece by piece in order to connect to these energies. You can also visualize the concept of a feeling, such as love and friendliness, empathy and concern, joy, enthusiasm or forgiveness. Visualizing meditation provides a means by which you can nurture positive emotions. But you can also visualize the image of a deity or mandala (a geometric pattern with abstract or concrete images), the picture of certain points or lines of force in your own body, or even events and situations, in order to unlock and experience the energies contained within them.

The classic meditation pose: Padmasana, the Lotus ▶

!

Meditation goes beyond study
Different kinds of meditation appeal to different people. Experiment to see which method suits you best, or depending on your individual situation, which is most appropriate to your needs.

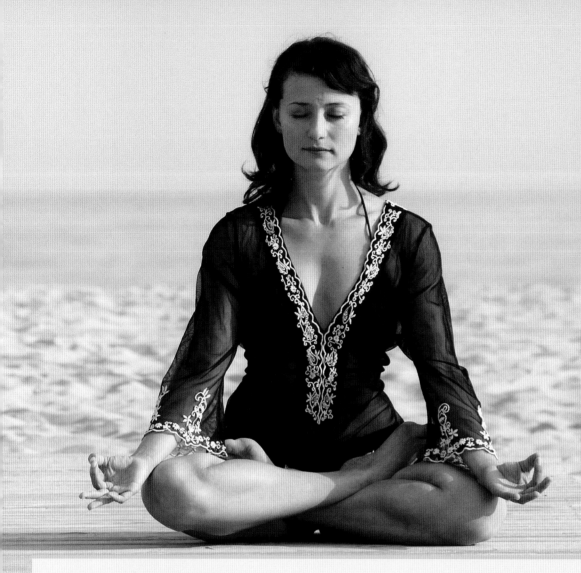

Instructions for meditation

There are lying, sitting and walking meditations, with seated meditation being the most popular and also the easiest to learn. The following classic meditation poses are ideal for ensuring that the spine remains straight and upright almost by itself (for instructions see pp.202–207):

- Egyptian Posture (see image p.226)
- Sukhasana, Easy Pose
- Siddhasana, Perfect Pose
- Virasana, Hero Pose
- Vajrasana, Thunderbolt
- (Ardha) Padmasana, (Half) Lotus

You should choose whichever position you feel happiest in, and one that is comfortable enough to remain in for the duration of the meditation, using a cushion or block if necessary. The meditation can last from five minutes and be increased depending upon the time you have available and how long you feel you need. At the beginning, any

position will probably become uncomfortable after a while, and your feet or legs may fall asleep; however, with a little practice, you will find that this soon passes. At the start of the meditation, you should take the following steps:

- Select your seating position.
- Close your eyes or focus on a point in the distance or on the floor.
- Lay your hands gently on your thighs, relax your leg, hip and buttock muscles and allow them to sink into the floor.
- Straighten your spine and draw your chin gently in towards your chest.
- First concentrate on your breath to become calm, and then on the object of your meditation (see pp.228–9).

Basically, you can meditate whenever, wherever and as long as you want, or are able to. However, it is advisable to make meditation a part of your daily or weekly routine, so that you can get used to it.

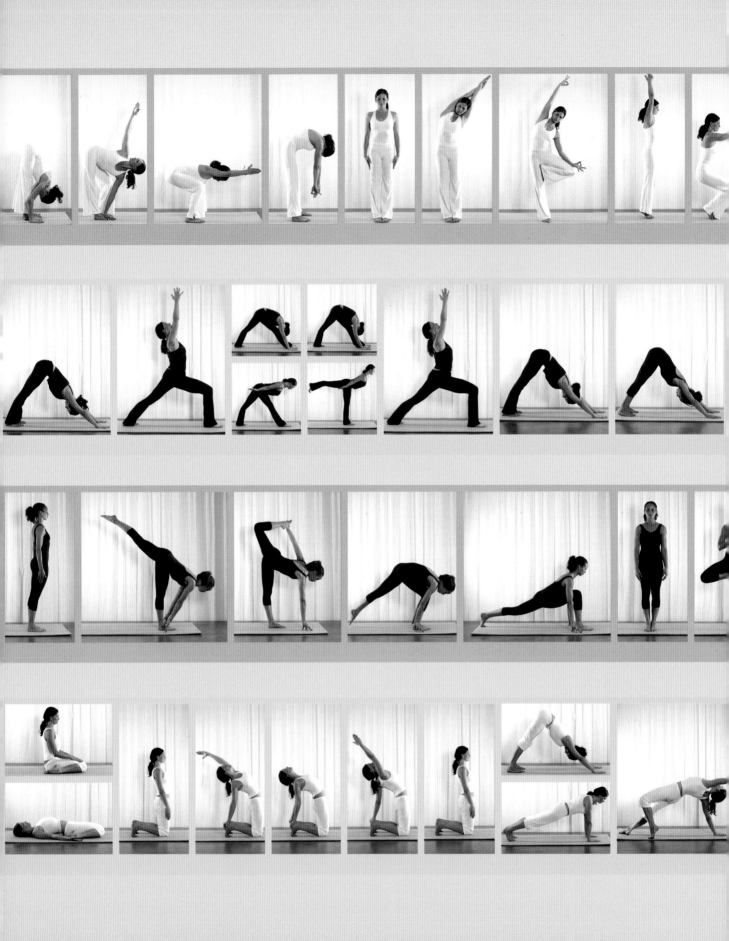

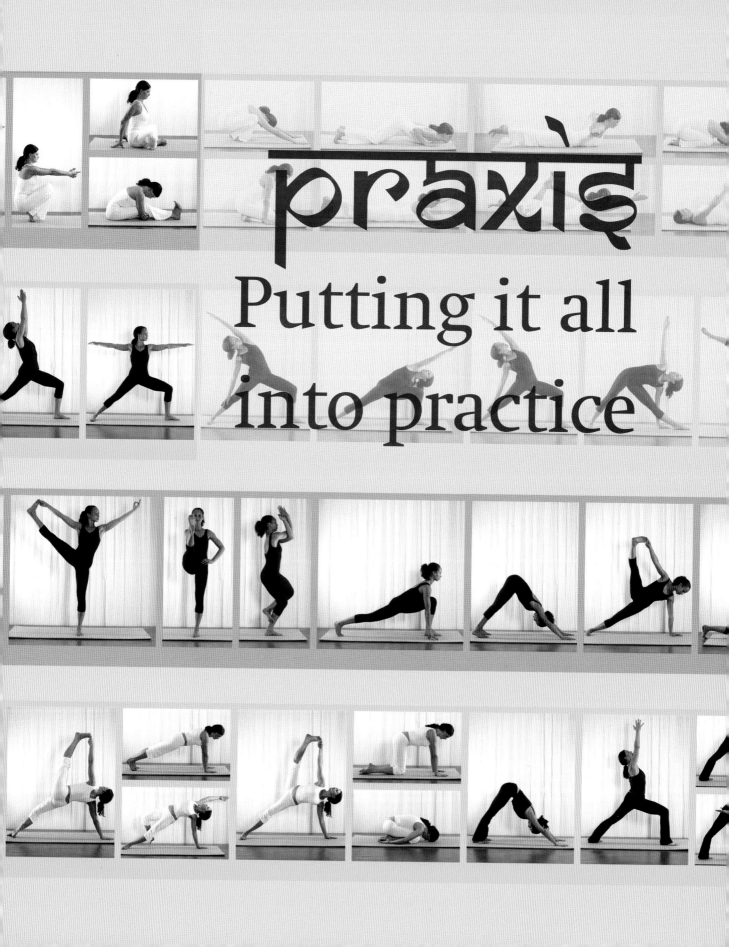

praxis
Putting it all into practice

Practical tips for asana practice, breathing exercises and meditation

Create an oasis for yourself

Whether you are practising asanas, pranayama, meditation or want to combine all three, you must first find a quiet place where you feel comfortable and where you are unlikely to be disturbed. If you mainly practise at home, create a small oasis of calm for yourself: arrange a corner in your house that you can keep clean and tidy, and decorate it with attractive objects such as candles, incense sticks and paintings or photographs.

The best time to practise

Traditionally, early morning is regarded as the ideal time to practise: this is when the mind is still calm and focused, the last meal was several hours ago and the body is well rested. But some people find practising in the morning difficult because their body often feels stiff. Apart from that, the various practice times and sequences have different effects, so depending on the time you have available, and what your needs and personal sensitivities are, you should experiment to find out what suits you best. The practice sequences on the following pages are all geared to these criteria, so you will find suggestions for various practice times and needs. Whatever you do, try to practise regularly, and ideally for a short time every day, rather than for a longer period only once a week.

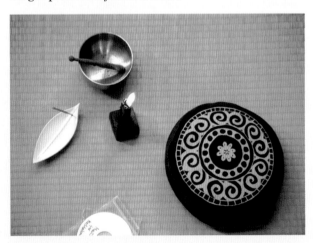

Many people find it easier to relax into meditation by playing gentle music, and burning candles and incense sticks.

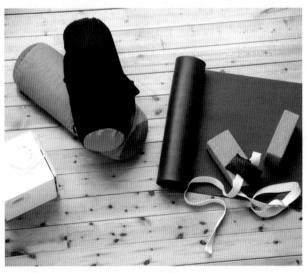

Before asana practice, make sure that any yoga props you may need – for example, a cushion, blocks or a belt – are within easy reach.

Perfect preparation

- Do not eat anything heavy for at least four hours or light snacks for at least two hours before your yoga practice.
- Wear comfortable, warm clothing – ideally several layers that are easy to take off once you have warmed up.
- Air the room where you are going to practise and make sure that it is at a pleasant temperature.
- Place any props, such as cushions, a blanket, belt and blocks, within easy reach.

Gentle start to yoga practice

Always start gently; adopt a comfortable sitting position, breathe naturally and first of all achieve inner calm. If you feel like it, practise a breathing exercise (see pp.220–23). Opinions differ on whether it is better to perform pranayama or meditation before or after asana practice. However, most people find it better to start with asana practice to calm the body and prepare it for the breathing exercises and meditation. Experiment to see what suits you best.

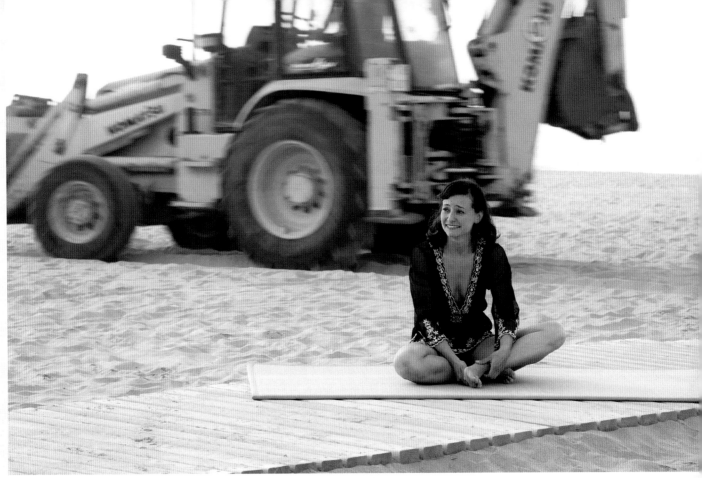

Choose a pleasant place for your yoga practice where – as far as possible – you are unlikely to be disturbed.

Observe yourself

As in so many things, practice makes perfect. When many people first take up yoga, they cannot imagine how they will ever be able to perform even the easiest-looking postures. But with a little patience, they soon become increasingly comfortable in the individual positions. Observe your body and respect its limits – do not force anything, but enjoy the growing sense of well-being that comes over you.

Exercise with caution

There are only a few restrictions for practising yoga, but here are some notes of advice that you should follow:

Do not practise:

- *if you are seriously ill or feeling exhausted;*
- *if you are suffering from acute pain.*

Be particularly careful with individual exercises, for example:

- *During menstruation, many teachers recommend that you do not practise any inverted postures, full bandhas or kapalbhati.*
- *Inverted postures are not recommended if you suffer from neck problems.*
- *In both the above cases, you should instead lie on the floor, let your back relax and stretch your legs up against a wall (see image p.237, bottom row, centre right).*

Take advice

- *In the case of chronic illness or recurring pain, yoga practice specifically targeted at these areas can have a healing or soothing effect. Consult your doctor and yoga teacher and put together your own tailor-made programme.*
- *There are special exercise programmes geared towards the specific needs of pregnant women, children and older people. Again, you should take advice and put together your own tailor-made programme.*

A fresh start to the day

The standing positions and backbends make this short practice sequence invigorating and provide you with energy for the whole day. It is recommended that you prepare yourself with warm-up exercises and two or three Sun Salutations (see pp.60–75).

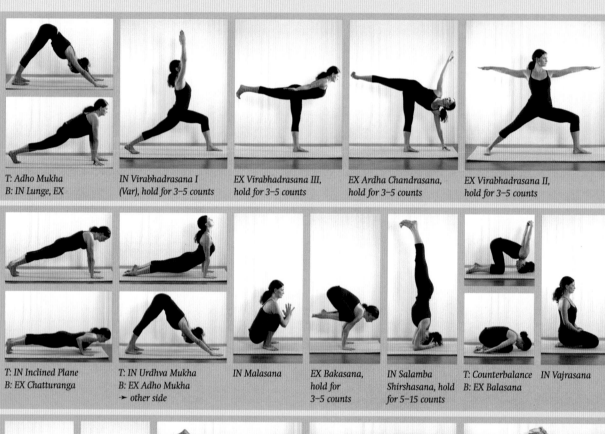

T: Adho Mukha
B: IN Lunge, EX

IN Virabhadrasana I (Var), hold for 3–5 counts

EX Virabhadrasana III, hold for 3–5 counts

EX Ardha Chandrasana, hold for 3–5 counts

EX Virabhadrasana II, hold for 3–5 counts

T: IN Inclined Plane
B: EX Chatturanga

T: IN Urdhva Mukha
B: EX Adho Mukha
→ other side

IN Malasana

EX Bakasana, hold for 3–5 counts

IN Salamba Shirshasana, hold for 5–15 counts

T: Counterbalance
B: EX Balasana

IN Vajrasana

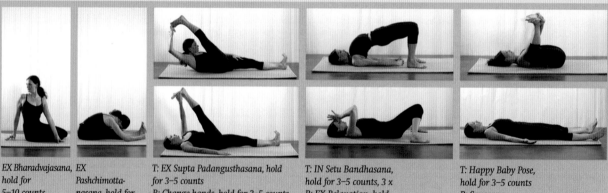

EX Bharadvajasana, hold for 5–10 counts

EX Pashchimotta-nasana, hold for 5–10 counts

T: EX Supta Padangusthasana, hold for 3–5 counts
B: Change hands, hold for 3–5 counts
→ other side

T: IN Setu Bandhasana, hold for 3–5 counts, 3 x
B: EX Relaxation, hold for 3–5 counts, 3 x

T: Happy Baby Pose, hold for 3–5 counts
B: Savasana

A peaceful end to the day

The floor positions and forward bends make this short practice sequence calming and relaxing – and allow you to fall asleep languorously. It is recommended that you start by preparing in the same way as for 'A fresh start to the day', but this is not absolutely necessary.

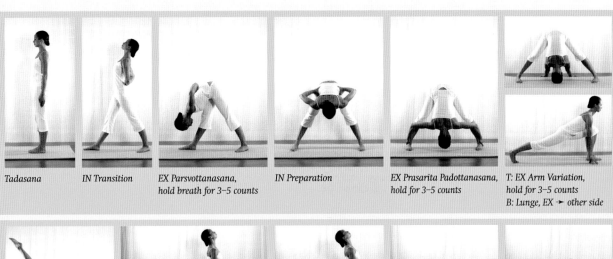

Tadasana

IN Transition

EX Parsvottanasana, hold breath for 3–5 counts

IN Preparation

EX Prasarita Padottanasana, hold for 3–5 counts

T: EX Arm Variation, hold for 3–5 counts
B: Lunge, EX ➤ other side

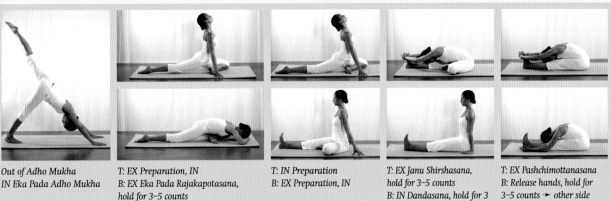

Out of Adho Mukha
IN Eka Pada Adho Mukha

T: EX Preparation, IN
B: EX Eka Pada Rajakapotasana, hold for 3–5 counts

T: IN Preparation
B: EX Preparation, IN

T: EX Janu Shirshasana, hold for 3–5 counts
B: IN Dandasana, hold for 3

T: EX Pashchimottanasana
B: Release hands, hold for 3–5 counts ➤ other side

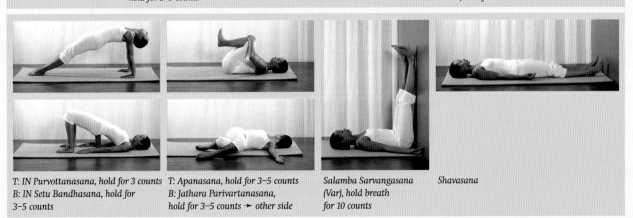

T: IN Purvottanasana, hold for 3 counts
B: IN Setu Bandhasana, hold for 3–5 counts

T: Apanasana, hold for 3–5 counts
B: Jathara Parivartanasana, hold for 3–5 counts ➤ other side

Salamba Sarvangasana (Var), hold breath for 10 counts

Shavasana

IN = inhale, EX = exhale, T: top photo, B: bottom photo, Var: Variation

Good for the back – in the morning

This short practice sequence is primarily aimed at strengthening the back muscles, but is also good for loosening and relaxing them. The standing positions and backbends make this a good sequence for the morning, since backbends in particular have an invigorating effect. If you have the time and energy, start with several warm-up exercises (see pp.56–9) and two or three Sun Salutations (see pp.60–75).

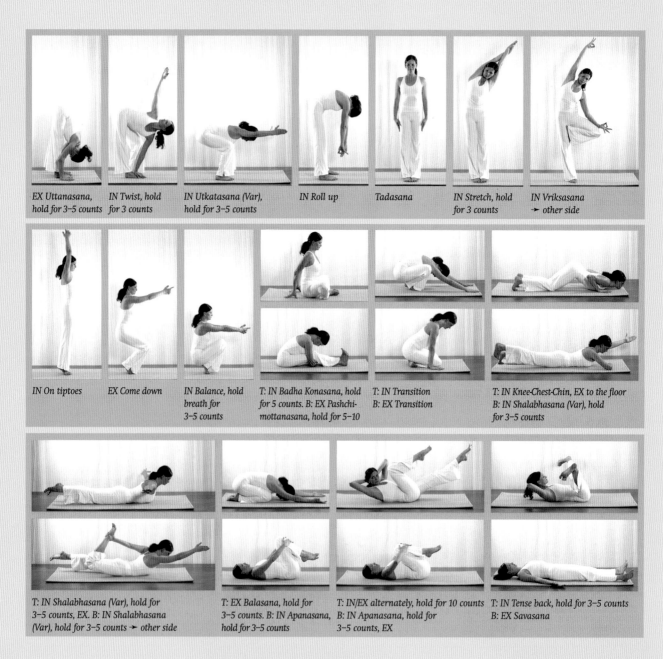

EX Uttanasana, hold for 3–5 counts

IN Twist, hold for 3 counts

IN Utkatasana (Var), hold for 3–5 counts

IN Roll up

Tadasana

IN Stretch, hold for 3 counts

IN Vriksasana → other side

IN On tiptoes

EX Come down

IN Balance, hold breath for 3–5 counts

T: IN Badha Konasana, hold for 5 counts. B: EX Pashchi-mottanasana, hold for 5–10

T: IN Transition B: EX Transition

T: IN Knee-Chest-Chin, EX to the floor B: IN Shalabhasana (Var), hold for 3–5 counts

T: IN Shalabhasana (Var), hold for 3–5 counts, EX. B: IN Shalabhasana (Var), hold for 3–5 counts → other side

T: EX Balasana, hold for 3–5 counts. B: IN Apanasana, hold for 3–5 counts

T: IN/EX alternately, hold for 10 counts B: IN Apanasana, hold for 3–5 counts, EX

T: IN Tense back, hold for 3–5 counts B: EX Savasana

Good for the back – in the evening

This sequence is suitable for the evening because it incorporates forward bends, which have a relaxing effect. It is also good for strengthening the back muscles, as well as for loosening and relaxing them.

Depending on how much time you have available and your energy levels, start with several warm-up exercises (see pp.56–9) and two or three Sun Salutations (see pp.60–75).

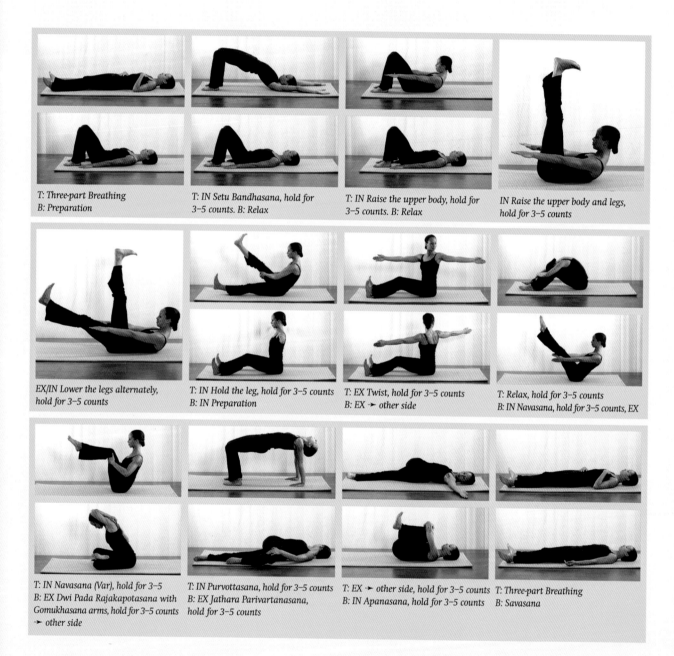

T: Three-part Breathing
B: Preparation

T: IN Setu Bandhasana, hold for 3–5 counts. B: Relax

T: IN Raise the upper body, hold for 3–5 counts. B: Relax

IN Raise the upper body and legs, hold for 3–5 counts

EX/IN Lower the legs alternately, hold for 3–5 counts

T: IN Hold the leg, hold for 3–5 counts
B: IN Preparation

T: EX Twist, hold for 3–5 counts
B: EX ➜ other side

T: Relax, hold for 3–5 counts
B: IN Navasana, hold for 3–5 counts, EX

T: IN Navasana (Var), hold for 3–5
B: EX Dwi Pada Rajakapotasana with Gomukhasana arms, hold for 3–5 counts ➜ other side

T: IN Purvottasana, hold for 3–5 counts
B: EX Jathara Parivartanasana, hold for 3–5 counts

T: EX ➜ other side, hold for 3–5 counts
B: IN Apanasana, hold for 3–5 counts

T: Three-part Breathing
B: Savasana

IN = inhale, EX = exhale, T: top photo, B: bottom photo, Var: Variation

Modular sequences

The following practice sequences are divided according to asana groups and level of difficulty, so that they can be combined with each other like a modular system.

This is how you use the modular system:

- Choose a sequence from each of the groups of standing positions, balance exercises, forward and backward bends, twists and inverted postures. You can of course combine various levels of difficulty.
- When making your selection, bear in mind the physiological and emotional effects of the exercises from the group of asanas and put your personal programme together according to your specific needs.
- At the start of a practice sequence, read the instructions for the individual positions carefully in the asana chapter, and if necessary use a yoga prop.

- Limber up using some of the warm-up exercises (see pp.56–9) and two or three Sun Salutations (see pp.60–75).
- Always finish your yoga practice with the Savasana relaxation position (see p.215). As a rule of thumb: ½ hour practice = approximately 3–5 minutes Savasana; 1 hour practice = 5–7 minutes Savasana; 1½ hours practice = 7–10 minutes Savasana.
- Depending upon the time you have and how you feel, combine asana practice with a breathing exercise (see pp.220–23), either before or afterwards, or end with a meditation – asana practice is perfect for preparing your body for this.

Standing positions

Physiological effects: These positions strengthen the foot, leg and torso muscles, stimulate blood circulation and expand the volume of the breath.

Emotional effects: These positions promote a feeling of being grounded, stability, endurance and stamina; they also strengthen self-awareness and inner security.

... for beginners

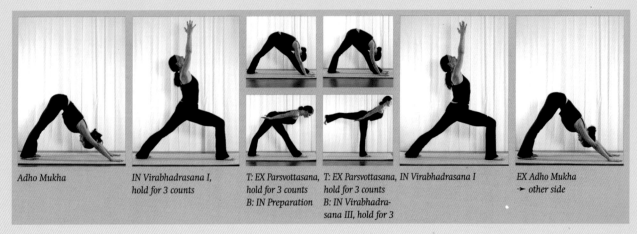

Adho Mukha

IN Virabhadrasana I, hold for 3 counts

T: EX Parsvottasana, hold for 3 counts
B: IN Preparation

T: EX Parsvottasana, hold for 3 counts
B: IN Virabhadra-sana III, hold for 3

IN Virabhadrasana I

EX Adho Mukha
➤ other side

... advanced exercises

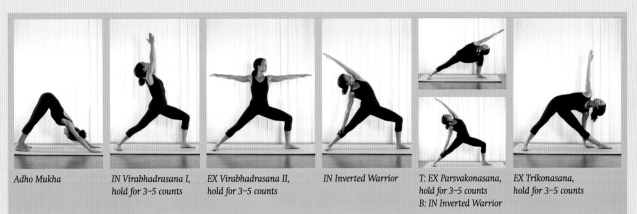

Adho Mukha

IN Virabhadrasana I,
hold for 3–5 counts

EX Virabhadrasana II,
hold for 3–5 counts

IN Inverted Warrior

T: EX Parsvakonasana,
hold for 3–5 counts
B: IN Inverted Warrior

EX Trikonasana,
hold for 3–5 counts

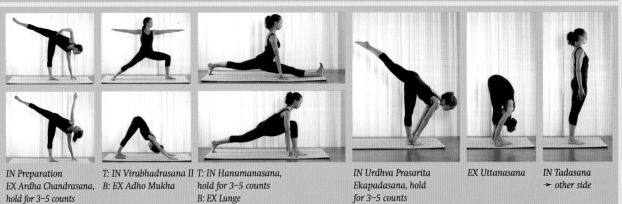

IN Preparation
EX Ardha Chandrasana,
hold for 3–5 counts

T: IN Virabhadrasana II
B: EX Adho Mukha

T: IN Hanumanasana,
hold for 3–5 counts
B: EX Lunge

IN Urdhva Prasarita
Ekapadasana, hold
for 3–5 counts

EX Uttanasana

IN Tadasana
➜ other side

... if you want to try something new

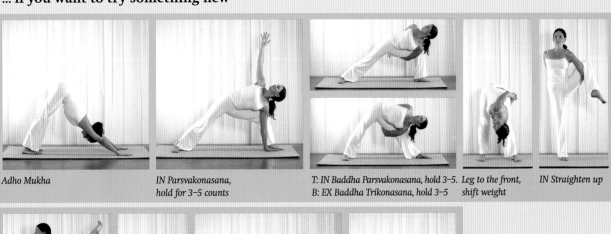

Adho Mukha

IN Parsvakonasana,
hold for 3–5 counts

T: IN Baddha Parsvakonasana, hold 3–5.
B: EX Baddha Trikonasana, hold 3–5

Leg to the front,
shift weight

IN Straighten up

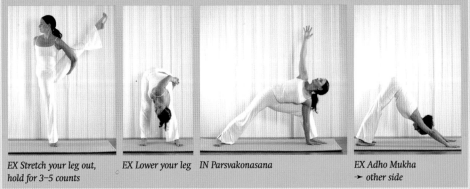

EX Stretch your leg out,
hold for 3–5 counts

EX Lower your leg

IN Parsvakonasana

EX Adho Mukha
➜ other side

IN = inhale, EX = exhale, T: top photo, B: bottom photo

Balance exercises

Physiological effects: These exercises strengthen the arm, shoulder, back, stomach and leg muscles. They also stimulate vital energy and improve the sense of balance.

Emotional effects: These postures stimulate the ability of the body and spirit to align to a common point. They also provide a feeling of balance and increase self-confidence.

... for beginners

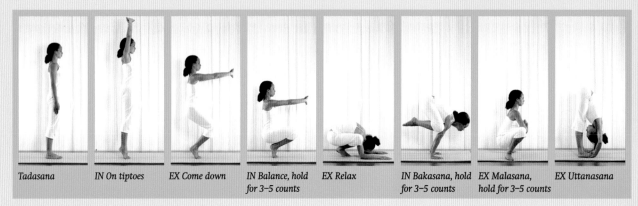

Tadasana

IN On tiptoes

EX Come down

IN Balance, hold for 3–5 counts

EX Relax

IN Bakasana, hold for 3–5 counts

EX Malasana, hold for 3–5 counts

EX Uttanasana

... advanced exercises

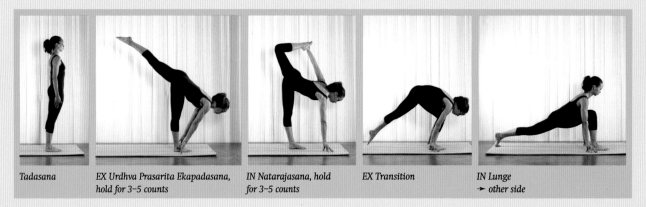

Tadasana

EX Urdhva Prasarita Ekapadasana, hold for 3–5 counts

IN Natarajasana, hold for 3–5 counts

EX Transition

IN Lunge
→ other side

... if you want to try something new

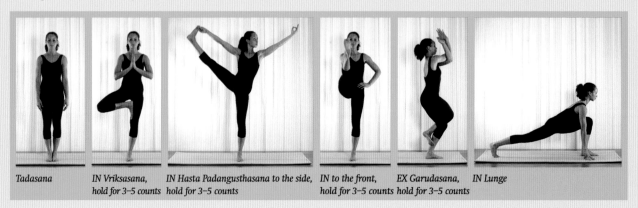

Tadasana

IN Vriksasana, hold for 3–5 counts

IN Hasta Padangusthasana to the side, hold for 3–5 counts

IN to the front, hold for 3–5 counts

EX Garudasana, hold for 3–5 counts

IN Lunge

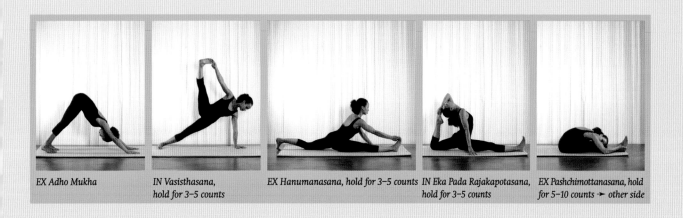

EX Adho Mukha

IN Vasisthasana, hold for 3–5 counts

EX Hanumanasana, hold for 3–5 counts

IN Eka Pada Rajakapotasana, hold for 3–5 counts

EX Pashchimottanasana, hold for 5–10 counts ➤ other side

Backbends

Physiological effects: They stretch and open the front of the body, particularly the chest area; they strengthen the back of the body, energize and invigorate.

Emotional effects: They open up the heart and improve feelings of trust in others. They also lighten the temperament.

... for beginners

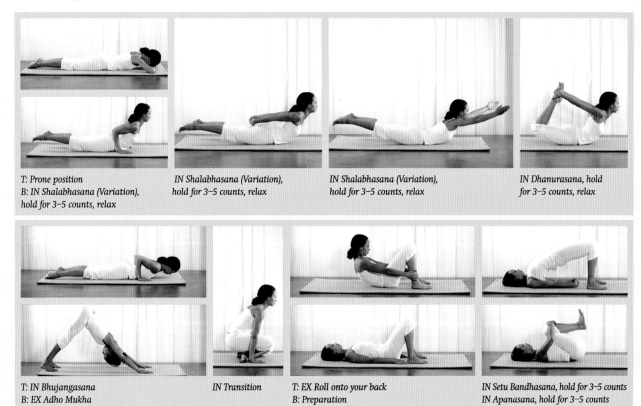

T: Prone position
B: IN Shalabhasana (Variation), hold for 3–5 counts, relax

IN Shalabhasana (Variation), hold for 3–5 counts, relax

IN Shalabhasana (Variation), hold for 3–5 counts, relax

IN Dhanurasana, hold for 3–5 counts, relax

T: IN Bhujangasana
B: EX Adho Mukha

IN Transition

T: EX Roll onto your back
B: Preparation

IN Setu Bandhasana, hold for 3–5 counts
IN Apanasana, hold for 3–5 counts

IN = inhale, EX = exhale, T: top photo, B: bottom photo

... advanced exercises

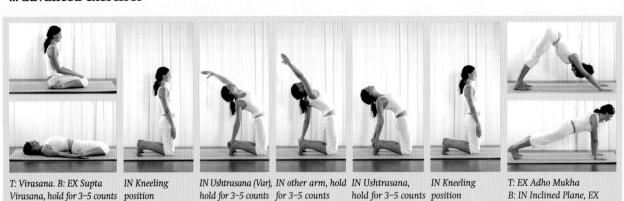

T: Virasana. B: EX Supta
Virasana, hold for 3–5 counts

IN Kneeling
position

IN Ushtrasana (Var),
hold for 3–5 counts

IN other arm, hold
for 3–5 counts

IN Ushtrasana,
hold for 3–5 counts

IN Kneeling
position

T: EX Adho Mukha
B: IN Inclined Plane, EX

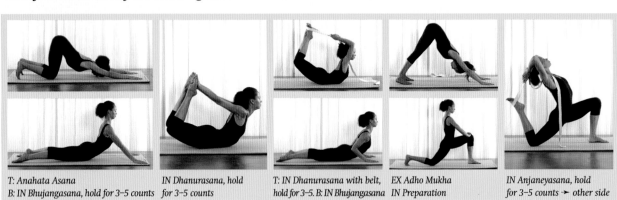

IN Preparation, hold for 3–5 counts

IN Vasisthasana, hold
for 3–5 counts

T: EX Inclined Plane
B: IN other side, hold for 3–5

IN Vasisthasana, other side
hold for 3–5 counts

T: EX All fours, hold for
3–5 counts. B: EX Balasana

... if you want to try something new

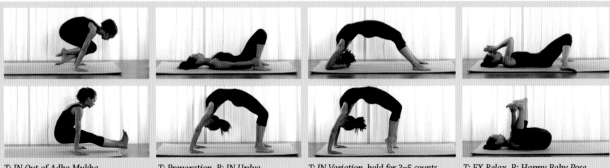

T: Anahata Asana
B: IN Bhujangasana, hold for 3–5 counts

IN Dhanurasana, hold
for 3–5 counts

T: IN Dhanurasana with belt,
hold for 3–5. B: IN Bhujangasana

EX Adho Mukha
IN Preparation

IN Anjaneyasana, hold
for 3–5 counts ➤ other side

T: IN Out of Adho Mukha
B: Jump through the legs

T: Preparation. B: IN Urdva
Dhanurasana, hold for 3–5 counts

T: IN Variation, hold for 3–5 counts
B: IN Urdva Dhanurasana, hold for 3–5

T: EX Relax. B: Happy Baby Pose,
hold for 3–5 counts

Forward bends

Physiological effects: They stretch the whole back of the body and create space in the waist, the groin, stomach and lower back.

Emotional effects: They have a calming effect, and they encourage relaxation and the ability to let go and overcome barriers.

... for beginners

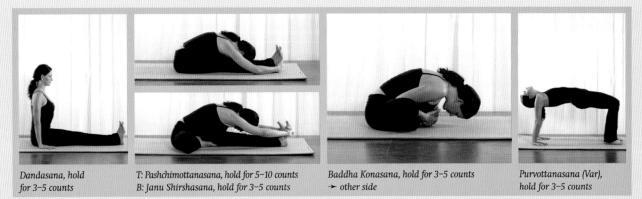

Dandasana, hold
for 3–5 counts

T: Pashchimottanasana, hold for 5–10 counts
B: Janu Shirshasana, hold for 3–5 counts

Baddha Konasana, hold for 3–5 counts
➤ other side

Purvottanasana (Var),
hold for 3–5 counts

... advanced exercises

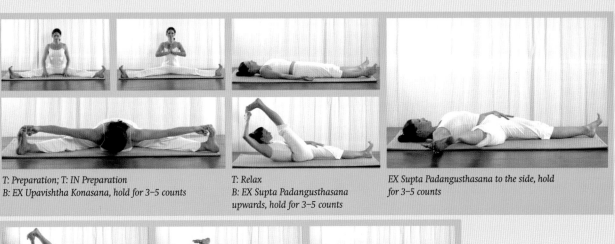

T: Preparation; T: IN Preparation
B: EX Upavishtha Konasana, hold for 3–5 counts

T: Relax
B: EX Supta Padangusthasana
upwards, hold for 3–5 counts

EX Supta Padangusthasana to the side, hold
for 3–5 counts

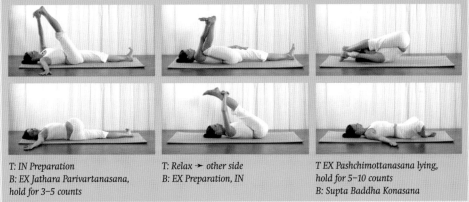

T: IN Preparation
B: EX Jathara Parivartanasana,
hold for 3–5 counts

T: Relax ➤ other side
B: EX Preparation, IN

T EX Pashchimottanasana lying,
hold for 5–10 counts
B: Supta Baddha Konasana

... if you want to try something new

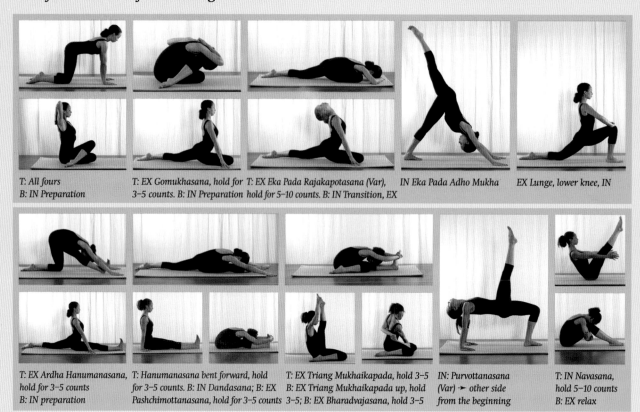

T: All fours
B: IN Preparation

T: EX Gomukhasana, hold for 3–5 counts. B: IN Preparation

T: EX Eka Pada Rajakapotasana (Var), hold for 5–10 counts. B: IN Transition, EX

IN Eka Pada Adho Mukha

EX Lunge, lower knee, IN

T: EX Ardha Hanumanasana, hold for 3–5 counts
B: IN preparation

T: Hanumanasana bent forward, hold for 3–5 counts. B: IN Dandasana; B: EX Pashchimottanasana, hold for 3–5 counts

T: EX Triang Mukhaikapada, hold 3–5
B: EX Triang Mukhaikapada up, hold 3–5; B: EX Bharadvajasana, hold 3–5

IN: Purvottanasana (Var) → other side from the beginning

T: IN Navasana, hold 5–10 counts
B: EX relax

Twists

Physiological effects: They help to cleanse and stimulate the digestive organs and regulate digestion. They also release tension and neutralize the spine.

Emotional effects: They help to develop the ability to remain calm and relaxed in tense situations.

... for beginners

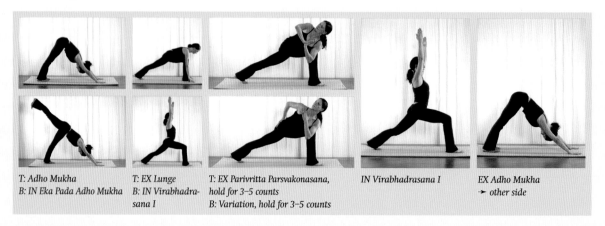

T: Adho Mukha
B: IN Eka Pada Adho Mukha

T: EX Lunge
B: IN Virabhadrasana I

T: EX Parivritta Parsvakonasana, hold for 3–5 counts
B: Variation, hold for 3–5 counts

IN Virabhadrasana I

EX Adho Mukha → other side

... advanced exercises

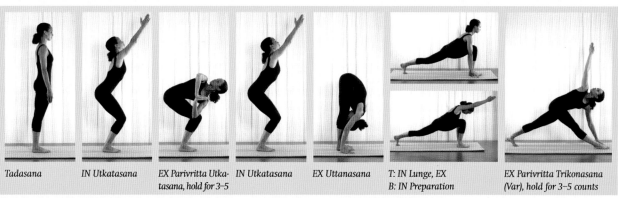

Tadasana

IN Utkatasana

EX Parivritta Utka-
tasana, hold for 3–5

IN Utkatasana

EX Uttanasana

T: IN Lunge, EX
B: IN Preparation

EX Parivritta Trikonasana
(Var), hold for 3–5 counts

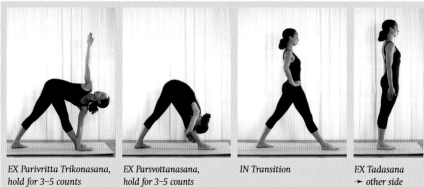

EX Parivritta Trikonasana,
hold for 3–5 counts

EX Parsvottanasana,
hold for 3–5 counts

IN Transition

EX Tadasana
➤ other side

... if you want to try something new

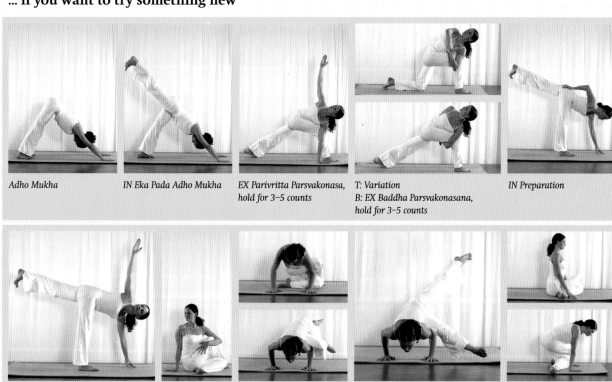

Adho Mukha

IN Eka Pada Adho Mukha

EX Parivritta Parsvakonasa,
hold for 3–5 counts

T: Variation
B: EX Baddha Parsvakonasana,
hold for 3–5 counts

IN Preparation

EX Parivritta Ardha Chandrasana,
hold for 3–5 counts

EX Ardha Matsyen-
drasana, hold 3–5

T: Preparation
B: Preparation

IN Eka Pada Koundinyasana I,
hold for 3–5 counts

T/B: Jump into Adho Mukhan
➤ other side

IN = inhale, EX = exhale, T: top photo, B: bottom photo, Var: Variation

Inverted postures

Physiological effects: They have a general 'rejuvenating' effect on the whole of the body: activating blood circulation, relieving the body's organs and providing the body with energy.

Emotional effects: These postures provide a feeling of stability and balance, and open up new perspectives, nurturing feelings of courage and the ability to overcome your fears.

... for beginners

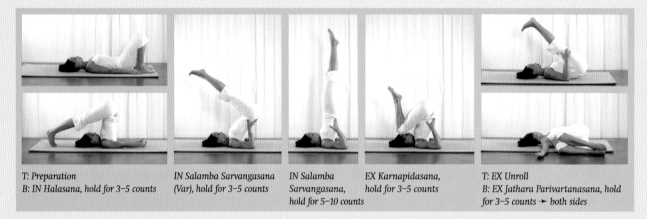

T: Preparation
B: IN Halasana, hold for 3–5 counts

IN Salamba Sarvangasana (Var), hold for 3–5 counts

IN Salamba Sarvangasana, hold for 5–10 counts

EX Karnapidasana, hold for 3–5 counts

T: EX Unroll
B: EX Jathara Parivartanasana, hold for 3–5 counts ➤ both sides

... advanced exercises I

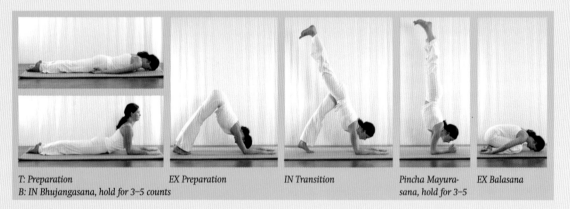

T: Preparation
B: IN Bhujangasana, hold for 3–5 counts

EX Preparation

IN Transition

Pincha Mayurasana, hold for 3–5

EX Balasana

... advanced exercises II

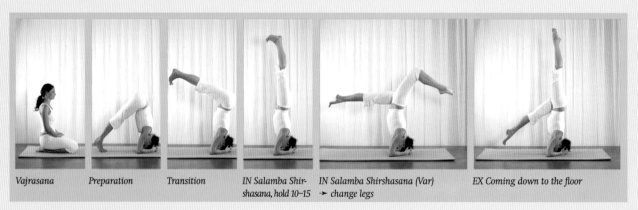

Vajrasana

Preparation

Transition

IN Salamba Shirshasana, hold 10–15

IN Salamba Shirshasana (Var) ➤ change legs

EX Coming down to the floor

... advanced exercises III

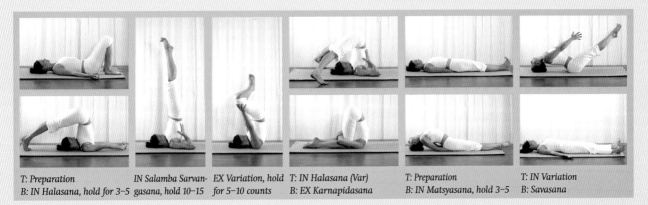

T: Preparation
B: IN Halasana, hold for 3–5

IN Salamba Sarvan-
gasana, hold 10–15

EX Variation, hold
for 5–10 counts

T: IN Halasana (Var)
B: EX Karnapidasana

T: Preparation
B: IN Matsyasana, hold 3–5

T: IN Variation
B: Savasana

.... if you want to try something new

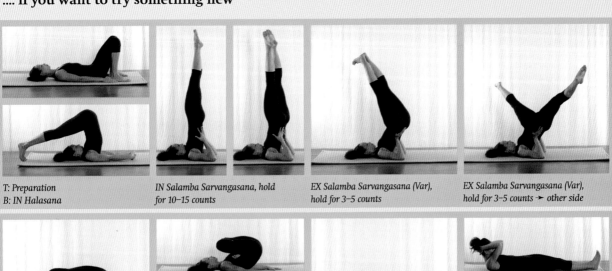

T: Preparation
B: IN Halasana

IN Salamba Sarvangasana, hold
for 10–15 counts

EX Salamba Sarvangasana (Var),
hold for 3–5 counts

EX Salamba Sarvangasana (Var),
hold for 3–5 counts ➤ other side

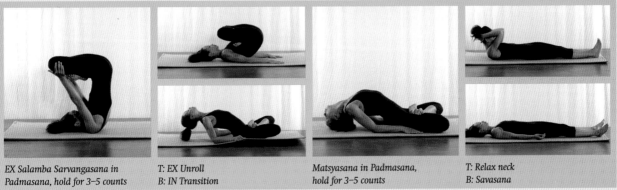

EX Salamba Sarvangasana in
Padmasana, hold for 3–5 counts

T: EX Unroll
B: IN Transition

Matsyasana in Padmasana,
hold for 3–5 counts

T: Relax neck
B: Savasana

IN = inhale, EX = exhale, T: top photo, B: bottom photo, Var: Variation

Glossary

Abhinivesha – the vague fear of the unknown, ultimately of death; one of the five ➤ Kleshas

Ahimsa – non-violence; one of the five ➤ Yamas

Aparigraha – non-covetousness; one of the five ➤ Yamas

Asana – the yogic body postures; the third stage of ➤ Patanjali's Ashtanga Marga

Ashtanga Marga – the Eight-Limb Path to enlightenment of ➤ Patanjali

Asmita – exaggerated egotism; one of the five ➤ Kleshas

Asteya – non-stealing; one of the five ➤ Yamas

Atman – the godly part of the inner self, in Indian philosophy the core essence of the individual

Avidya – lack of knowledge (ignorance) or incorrect knowledge; one of the five ➤ Kleshas

Bandha – internal body lock to control the flow of ➤ Prana

Bhagavad Gita – literally 'The Song of God'; one of the fundamental texts of yogic philosophy – besides ➤ Patanjali's Yoga Sutras and the ➤ Hatha Yoga Pradipika, part of the ➤ Mahabharata

Bhakti Yoga – yoga of love and devotion, and one of the five main paths of traditional yoga

Brahma – the creator, one of the three most important Indian gods – besides ➤ Shiva and ➤ Vishnu

Brahmacharya – moderation; one of the five ➤ Yamas

Brahmin – priest caste in India

Chakras – energy centres in the body associated with different qualities and characteristics; part of the anatomy in ➤ Hatha Yoga

Dharana – concentration; the sixth stage of ➤ Patanjali's Ashtanga Marga

Dharma – central concept of the Indian religion and philosophy: the destiny of mankind

Dhyana – meditation, the seventh stage of ➤ Patanjali's Ashtanga Marga

Dvesha – hatred; one of the five ➤ Kleshas

Guru – literally 'one who leads people from darkness to light'; master, teacher

Hatha Yoga – physical yoga, based on the ➤ Hatha Yoga Pradipika; one of the five main paths of traditional yoga

Hatha Yoga Pradipika – the fundamental text of ➤ Hatha Yoga

Ishvarapranidhana – trust in a higher power; one of the five ➤ Niyamas

Jnana Yoga – yoga of wisdom and knowledge; one of the five main paths of traditional yoga

Karma – cycle of cause and effect

Karma Yoga – yoga of selfless action; one of the five main paths of traditional yoga

Kleshas – afflictions of the mind

Koshas – astral and physical layers of the body to which various levels of consciousness are attributed; part of the anatomy in ➤ Hatha Yoga

Kundalini – according to Tantric teaching, the cosmic energy (➤ Shakti) that is present in all people and which yoga can activate in order to unite it with the divine consciousness (➤ Shiva)

Mahabharata – one of the most important Indian narrative works (besides the Ramayana), dating back to 500 BC; contains the ➤ Bhagavad Gita

Mantra – a syllable, word or phrase used in meditation

Maya – illusion, veil of perception

Mudra – certain bodily postures that channel the flow of ➤ Prana

Nadis – channels of energy within the body through which ➤ Prana circulates; part of the anatomy in ➤ Hatha Yoga

Nadi shodhana – breathing exercise for inner cleansing and harmonizing of the ➤ Nadis

Niyamas – personal rules of conduct; second stage of ➤ Patanjali's Ashtanga Marga

Patanjali – compiler of the ➤ Yoga Sutras, which form the basis of ➤ Raja Yoga – also called Classic Yoga (written between 200 BC and 200 AD)

Prana – life energy, circulates in the ➤ Nadis; part of the anatomy in ➤ Hatha Yoga

Pranayama – the channelling of energy through controlled breathing exercises; the fourth stage of ➤ Patanjali's Ashtanga Marga

Pratyahara – the withdrawal of the senses; the fifth stage of ➤ Patanjali's Ashtanga Marga

Raga – exaggerated attachment to pleasurable things, avarice; one of the five ➤ Kleshas

Raja Yoga – literally 'Yoga of the Kings', also called Classic Yoga, based on Patanjali's ➤ Yoga Sutras, the yogic spiritual path; one of the five main paths of traditional yoga

Sadhu – in India a holy man, a sage, who has devoted himself to a religious, and in some cases, strictly ascetic life

Samadhi – the goal of yoga, which is a state of bliss, unification and enlightenment; the eighth stage of ➤ Patanjali's Ashtanga Marga

Samskara – deep-seated patterns of thought, conditioning and habits

Sanskrit – literally 'joined together', language of the Vedas and classical Indian culture

Santosha – contentment; one of the five ➤ Niyamas

Sat-chit-ananda – literally 'existence-consciousness-bliss' ➤ Samadhi

Satya – truthfulness; one of the five ➤ Yamas

Saucha – purity; one of the five ➤ Niyamas

Shakti – cosmic energy and power in every individual

Shiva – a) cosmic/divine awareness (as counterpart of ➤ Shakti, the cosmic energy of the individual); b) the destroyer, one of the most important Indian gods, besides ➤ Vishnu and ➤ Brahma; c) god of the yogis

Sutra – literally a 'string' or 'thread' in Indian literature ➤ Yoga Sutras

Svadhyaya – self-study, self-reflection; one of the five ➤ Niyamas

Swami – (Hindi) form of address for a scholar or religious teacher

Tantrism – an Indian religious movement (dating back to the 5th century) that significantly influenced the development of ➤ Hatha Yoga

Tapas – self-discipline; one of the five ➤ Niyamas

Trimurti – divine Trinity of ➤ Brahma ➤ Vishnu and ➤ Shiva

Upanishads – religious and philosophical fundamental texts in Sanskrit

Veda(s) – literally 'knowledge', the most ancient of India's fundamental religious texts

Vishnu – the maintainer, one of the three most important Indian gods besides ➤ Shiva and ➤ Brahma

Yamas – code of conduct for harmonizing external interactions in one's life, the first stage in ➤ Patanjali's Ashtanga Marga

Yoga – one of India's six major philosophical systems, the path to enlightenment

Yoga Sutras – fundamental text of ➤ Raja Yoga, compiled by ➤ Patanjali

Yogi – male practitioner of yoga

Acknowledgements

I would like to thank Lutz, Esther and Thierry of Parragon for giving
me the opportunity to write this book; Günther for the fantastic photographs
and his sensitivity in working with human subjects; Constanze, Dulce, Eduardo,
Nicole and Ijeoma for their enthusiasm and unstinting encouragement;
Last, but not least, I would like to thank my fantastic teachers who opened
up the world of yoga to me, and Frank for his unwavering mental support.

Index of names and subjects

Asanas and pranayama

Translation of body postures and breathing exercises

Bibliography

Appleton, K. *Yoga in Practice*. London: Macmillan 2004

Desikachar, T.K.V. *Health, Healing and Beyond*. New York: Aperture 2004

Desikachar, T.K.V. *The Heart of Yoga. Developing a Personal Practice*. Vermont: Inner Traditions 1999

Desikachar, T.K.V. *Über Freiheit und Meditation. Das Yoga-Sutra des Patanjali*. Petersberg: Via Nova 2003

Feuerstein, Georg and Payne, Larry *Yoga For Dummies*. New Jersey: John Wiley & Sons 1999

Gannon, Sharon and Life, David *Jivamukti Yoga*. New York: Ballantine Books 2002

Hawley, J. (Ed). *The Bhagavad Gita. A Walkthrough for Westerners*. Novato: New World Library 2001

Iyengar, B.K.S. *Iyengar Yoga For Beginners*. London: Dorling Kindersley 2006

Iyengar, B.K.S. *Light on Pranayama: The Yogic Art of Breathing*. New York: Crossroad Publishing Co. 2001

Iyengar, B.K.S. *Light on Yoga*. London: Thorsons 2001

Iyengar, B.K.S. *Yoga – Der Weg zu Gesundheit und Harmonie*. Munich: Dorling Kindersley 2001

Lark, L. *Yoga For Life*. London: Carlton Books 2001

Metha, M. *How to Use Yoga: A Step-by-step Guide to the Iyengar Method of Yoga, for Relaxation, Health and Well-Being*. London: Southwater 2006

Metha, M. *Yoga Explained*. London: Kyle Cathie Limited 2004

Osho. *Das Yogabuch. Die Geburt des Individuums*. Zürich: Innenwelt Verlag 2002

Saraswati, S. *Asana, Pranayama, Mudra and Bandha*. India: Bihar School of Yoga 2003

Stone, M. *The Inner Tradition of Yoga: A Guide to Yoga Philosophy for the Contemporary Practitioner*. Boston: Shambhala Publications Inc. 2008

Swatmarama, S. *Hatha Yoga Pradipika*. Charleston: Forgotten Books 2008

Trökes, A. *Hatha-Yoga-Pradipika. Eine Abhandlung über Hatha-Yoga*. Berlin: Eigenverlag 2006

Usharbudh, A. *Philosophy of Hatha Yoga*. Honnesdale, PA: Himalayan Institute Press 1989

Picture credits

Quotations

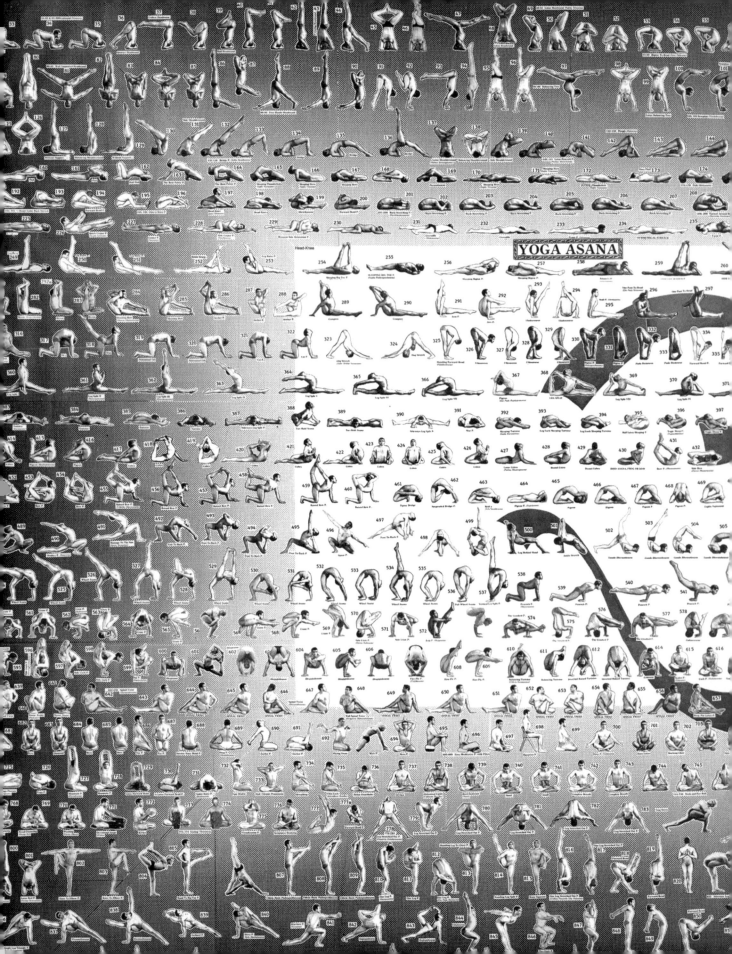

YOGA ASANA